T0315829

Handbook for Beginning
Mental Health Researchers

About the Editors

Peter Hauri, PhD, is Co-Director of both the Dartmouth Sleep Disorder Center and the Dartmouth Behavioral Medicine Section. He teaches graduate and undergraduate level classes at Dartmouth College, New Hampshire. Dr. Hauri is a nationally and internationally recognized expert on insomnia and sleep disorders.

Charlotte Sanborn, BPhD, is Director of the Faculty/Employee Assistance Program at Dartmouth College. She earned a BPhD degree in Behavioral Philosophy of Mental Health from the Pacific Western University. Her most recent research and clinical interest is in young adult suicide. She is President of the American Association of Suicidology, and a consulting editor for the *Journal of Suicide and Life Threatening Behavior*.

John Corson, PhD, is Professor of Psychiatry at Dartmouth Medical School, Adjunct Professor of Psychology at Dartmouth College, and Chief Psychologist at the White River Junction, Vermont Veterans Administration Hospital. He is the author of many publications on the topics of learning theory, stress, and psychophysiology.

Jeffrey Violette, MD, is former psychiatrist at the Community Health Counseling Services in Dover-Foxcroft, Maine. He completed his pathology residency at the Medical Center Hospital of Vermont and his psychiatry residency at Dartmouth Hitchcock Medical Center.

Handbook for Beginning Mental Health Researchers

Peter Hauri
Charlotte Sanborn
John Corson
Jeffrey Violette

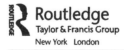
Routledge
Taylor & Francis Group
New York   London

Routledge is an imprint of the
Taylor & Francis Group, an informa business

Reprinted 2009 by Routledge

LIBRARY OF CONGRESS
Library of Congress Cataloging-in-Publication Data

Handbook for beginning mental health researchers / Peter Hauri . . . [et al.].
    p. cm.
  Bibliography: p.
  Includes index.
  ISBN 0-86656-719-4
  1. Psychiatry — Research — Methodology — Handbooks, manuals, etc. 2. Psychology —
Research — Methodology — Handbooks, manuals, etc. I. Hauri, Peter.
  [DNLM: 1. Mental Health. 2. Research — methods. WM 105 H2354]
RC337.H36   1988
616.89'027 — dc19
DNLM/DLC
for Library of Congress   87-35377
                                                                                            CIP

CONTENTS

Acknowledgements

We wish to gratefully acknowledge the contributions of the people listed below in alphabetical order, as well as the help of many other persons who may have contributed to this book and are not specifically named:

Percy Ballantine, MD
Assistant Professor
  of Clinical Psychiatry
  and Clinical Surgery
  (Neurosurgery)
Brattleboro Retreat
Brattleboro, VT

Walter E. Barton, MD
Professor of Psychiatry,
  Emeritus
Department of Psychiatry
Dartmouth Medical School
Hanover, NH

Jean Kinney, MSW
Assistant Professor of
  Clinical Psychiatry
Executive Director,
  Project Cork Institute
Dartmouth Medical School
Hanover, NH

Robert Landeen, MD
Department of Psychiatry
  and Behavioral Science
Stanford University
  School of Medicine
Stanford, CA

Henry Payson, MD, MSL
Professor of Clinical
  Psychiatry
Dartmouth Medical School
Hanover, NH

Trevor R. P. Price, MD
Associate Professor
Department of Psychiatry
University of Pennsylvania
  School of Medicine
Philadelphia, PA

Virginia Rolett
Director, Project Cork
    Resource Center
Dartmouth Medical School
Hanover, NH

Peter M. Silberfarb, MD
Professor of Psychiatry
    and Medicine
Chairman, Department of
    Psychiatry
Hanover, NH

Gregory B. Teague, PhD
Assistant Professor of
    Clinical Psychiatry
    (Psychology)
West Central Services
Hanover, NH

Gary J. Tucker, MD
Professor and Chairman
Department of Psychiatry
    and Behavioral Sciences
University of Washington
Dartmouth Medical School
Seattle, WA

Foreword

The need for a beginner's manual in mental health research has been filled by the team of Hauri, Sanborn, Corson and Violette. They share their experience gained through years of active research and teaching of both psychiatric residents and psychology students starting careers in the mental health professions. The authors have set down the fundamentals for beginning a research project in a simple, clearly written manual.

Essential to good clinical practice is a research attitude that constantly evaluates what we think we know. We observe the patient, adjust the treatment as needed, evaluate the response, and explore for facts.

Readers of this book will learn to formulate a clear hypothesis, select a representative population, conduct a valid study, and clearly describe results and conclusions. Most of what we learn becomes obsolete in a short time with the swift advance of science. To keep abreast, we read the literature. To discover truth in the mass of reported research, critical judgment is necessary. Without a research attitude and a critical sense in reading literature, clinical practice can suffer.

After explaining why all psychiatric residents, social workers and psychology students preparing for the mental health professions should acquire a research attitude, the authors discuss how mental health research is done. The varieties of research are described from anecdotal case reports, to studies with few variables, to complex investigation of multiple variables. The need for careful observation, meticulous records, and diligent, obsessive attention to detail is explained.

In a chapter on how to do research the authors describe the basic research procedures as: (1) a clear definition of an area of focus, reviewing what others have done on the same issue; (2) thinking about the problem and determining the specific hypothesis to be tested, (3) selecting the method to be used to find the answer to the question posed, (4) planning the data gathering process, (5) execution of the project and analysis of data, and (6) communicating the results to others.

The authors point out that central to choosing any research project is the answer to the question I call, "So what?" When the project is completed, what will it accomplish? Will it increase awareness of a problem? Expand knowledge? Advance science? In answering these questions, one should consider the responsibility of a mental health professional to society and to its values and ethics.

This book is an insightful exposition of the fundamental factors essential to good research. It is a useful guide for every beginner in mental health research.

Walter E. Barton, MD
Dartmouth Medical School

Introduction

This handbook arises out of the strong conviction that our clinical work almost always benefits if we do some research as well. We believe that it is essential to good clinical practice in mental health to have an open mind, a searching, critical attitude, and a hard-nosed, careful evaluation of what we do know, and what we do not know. We know of no better way to nurture and foster these desirable clinical attributes than to engage in careful, publishable research.

One important message of our book is a strong belief that it is not all that difficult to do good mental health research. Sure, it is not child's play! It has its own codes, rituals, and procedures that need to be mastered. This is what our book is trying to teach. However, in the long run, most research procedures and codes are simply variants of common sense. Doing good research, we believe, is no more difficult than doing good clinical work.

The extent to which we incorporate a research attitude and bring an inquiring and critical mind to our work is the extent to which we have grown from simple technicians into the role of true professionals. To rise above the technician level is often difficult because many training programs emphasize mostly how to do things, with little attention paid to a critical appraisal of why we are doing things that way. Hopefully, working on research will help asking the "whys" instead of the "how to's."

This book has a history. As most others, our Psychiatry Department at Dartmouth runs research seminars for mental health workers (psychiatric residents, psychology interns, social workers, nurses). Most of the chapters in this book started as lecture notes for these seminars, or as handouts. Over the last decade the instructors in these seminars varied, and each expanded and rewrote what the predecessor had done. Finally, this resulted in a mimeographed handbook, planned for internal consumption only. Others saw our handbook, liked it, and encouraged us to make it more widely available. Thus, our handbook has the advantage of being field tested and revised, based on our experiences during many seminars and based on feedback from our students. The first three authors of this book are simply those three of us who took what had been written over the years by them and by others (mentioned in the acknowledgements) and put it into a more uniform structure.

Jeff Violette, our last author, is a graduate of our program and a psychiatrist who has managed to publish repeatedly during his residency. First we had simply asked Jeff to critique our work. Cooperation developed, and he finished by writing our last chapter. He is a living example of how much can be done with little time and little money.

We feel that our book can be used in seminars, but that it also can be studied by the individual who wants to, or needs to, develop research skills on his/her own. The book probably should be read twice. Read it first at a more superficial level to get a feeling for what may be involved in research. Then read it again, slowly this time, chapter by chapter, and ask yourself some of the questions that we suggest. You may be surprised. By the time you have worked yourself through the first half of our book for the second time, you might be well on your way to your first publication.

Research is often viewed with ambivalence. Laymen and professionals alike believe that research endeavors are basically worthwhile. Yet, despite these good feelings about it, the actual number of professionals who engage in research is small. Perhaps the simplest explanation for this disparity between lip services to research and actually doing it is the way research activities are taught to trainees. To students, research is often a requirement, an enforced activity; or the student is presented with the model of a researcher who inhabits a large laboratory, peopled by many technicians doing obviously highly technical tasks. Also, the research findings that are presented to students often seem so complex and so far removed from any practical application that students feel they would have to give up most anything else to be a researcher. Although such opinions are widely held, they are wrong, as we try to show in this book.

Courses on research for mental health trainees frequently become courses in how impossible research is in mental health matters. There is more emphasis on the pitfalls and problems of research than on the positive aspects of it. Certainly, the number of variables that can affect behavioral research is almost infinite, and it is easy to make mistakes in this field. So what? Just because nobody has yet done a perfect piece of research does not mean that research should stop. Also, because most researchers are somewhat compulsive, this is often conveyed to the trainees. Instead of undertaking a "do-able" research project, the trainees then spend most of their time designing the impossible "perfect study." All of this seems unnecessary and unfortunate.

Let us briefly examine the goals for research, as developed by the President's Biomedical Research Panel in 1976. This panel developed the following six goals for biomedical research.

1. Discovery, through research, of new knowledge and the relating of new knowledge to the existing base;
2. Translation of new knowledge, through applied research, into new technology and strategy for health care;
3. Validation of new technology through clinical trials;
4. Determination of the safety and efficacy of new technology through demonstration projects;
5. Education of the professional community in the proper use of the new technology and of the lay community in the nature of these developments; and
6. Skillful and balanced application of the new developments to the population.

We can readily see that these goals not only portray the researcher as the developer of new knowledge but also as the applicant of new knowledge to a clinical population. Not all researchers are involved in generating new knowledge at the bench.

True, to finish a piece of research takes considerable determination. Many hours of boredom and routine work are inevitable in any study, however exciting it might seem to be at the onset and however interesting its final form. Nevertheless, the satisfaction of finishing a piece of work is great indeed, and it is within the grasp of many more people than at present undertake research in mental health. The harvest is truly great, and the laborers are few, so — have a go!

Chapter 1

Why Should You Do
Mental Health Research?

We define the research attitude as a frame of mind that constantly re-evaluates what we think we know, speculates on mental health issues, and then develops ways to test these speculations. Such a research attitude is not only crucial to the acquisition of new knowledge, it appears to be essential for enlightened clinical practice as well.

Good research adds a permanent new piece to our knowledge of the universe. Good mental health research discovers new facts or relationships in the area of mental health. Such work adds new pieces to the puzzle that we are trying to put together concerning the facts and the laws of human functioning. Once discovered, each new research piece of the puzzle is expected to remain solid until the end of time. It is an exhilarating experience to work in research in mental health, and it is exciting to contribute something that will remain permanently in place long after we all have died. Note that we are not talking here about the narcissistic desire to get one's own name on some piece of a disease or a theory, or to build oneself a monument. Rather, we are talking about the healthy human desire to use one's life in the pursuit of something that may be of lasting benefit.

Poor research is worse than nothing. It misleads others who work in the area. It is better not to know anything in a certain mental health area and to start from scratch rather than to assume we know certain facts, build on them, and then have the whole edifice crumble because the foundations were poor. It is imperative that if we do research, we do it well.

Although the goal of all research is the discovery of permanent knowledge, if research were done only for this goal, we could leave the task to a few large research institutions and a few intellectual giants. The message of this book is that such a course of events would be a disaster. We feel that every good clinician should do some research, because the research attitude gained from it is indispensable for good clinical work as well. We define the research attitude as a frame of mind that is constantly re-evaluating what we think we know, is always speculating on how our minds and our treatments work, and is then developing ways to test these speculations.

To do research, we need to know about certain issues and tools. For example, we need to know about control groups; we need to know how much the bias of an observer can influence what he sees; we need to know about probabilities and ways to assess whether what we observe is actually caused by what we did. Might the effects we see be due to some other factor or to chance fluctuations? This book discusses some of these tools and tries to get you started on doing some research.

Sainsbury and Kreitman (1975) have addressed themselves to the question "why do research?" as follows:

> The most important value of research, however, is that it is not only research into the outside world but also research into oneself. It is learning to acquire critical judgement, not only of the works of others, but also in the evaluation of one's own abilities. Through it one should acquire the habit of constant checking on the validity of everyday clinical practice. For example, are your routine drug regimens for depression and other psychiatric illnesses up to date and still effective? . . . Do you listen to patients carefully, and is there a proper feedback to you of your junior's critical comments on your ideas and practices? A little healthy skepticism about one's clinical skill is all the more effective if it results in an investigation to confirm or deny doubts.

The practitioners of medicine were probably as intelligent in past centuries as they are today. Yet little progress was made in their treatment of disease until fairly recently because these practitioners lacked the tools of research. They cared little about double-blind control groups, double-blind outcome studies, the statistical evaluation of what might be caused by chance, or contaminating factors. No doubt these practitioners of yesteryear were excellent clinicians. They treated their patients as they had learned from their elders. They observed what happened. And they assumed, often erroneously, that what they had done to the patient had caused that outcome. Over the years, we probably could have avoided many serious errors had previous clinicians known about the tools of research. Would we have applied leeches to sick people for as long as we did, had a research attitude permeated clinical work at that time? Could Kraepelin, brilliant as he was, have stampeded us into warehousing millions of schizophrenics for their entire lives, had clinicians used a research attitude and more carefully evaluated his claim that we were dealing with incurable premature senility? No telling what similar foibles we commit today. But we shall overcome our current mistakes faster if clinicians bring a research attitude to each client encounter, aware of how biased their own observations can often be, and striving to remain critical and to give alternative hypotheses a chance to prove themselves.

Today we are flooded with new information. How are we to deal with this knowledge explosion unless we have learned to separate the wheat from the chaff? Without this critical evaluation, we can only become bloated from too much new input (because we believe it all), or we can stagnate because we have stopped reading (it was too much to absorb), or we can become cynical.

How does one foster a research attitude? We know of no better way than to involve ourselves directly in the active and critical generation of new knowledge, i.e., to do research ourselves. To carry through a research project tempers the mind, and we look at our knowledge in a different way.

In discussing the exhilaration and the excitement when research has paid off for you, we do not want to belittle the obstacles. To finish a piece of research work takes considerable determination. Also, many hours of boredom and routine work are inevitable in every study, no matter how exciting in conception and no matter how interesting its final outcome will be.

In the recent past, there have been dramatic ups and downs both in research optimism and in research support. The National Institute of Mental Health awarded its first research grants as late as 1948. Mental health research has rapidly expanded since then. It has provided us with increasingly sophisticated information and new ideas about causes, treatments, and preventions of psychological problems. Brown (1977) noted that such research is essential to the continuing development of mental health procedures and resources. However, after some decades of almost unlimited optimism regarding what research can bring, we seem to be now in a period of more limited expectations both about what research can do and what research monies can buy. Brown (1977) worries that those who might have had a desire to pursue a career in mental health research will now turn their energies elsewhere. "Today the impact is felt in a stagnation of knowledge development; tomorrow it will tell in a paucity of experienced researchers. . . . "

Finances and available time do limit the scope of what can be done, but they do not eliminate the need for each of us to develop a research attitude. Although research is easier when money flows freely, much research can be done on limited budgets. An important objective of this handbook is to describe the range of research possibilities and to point out what a beginner without money can do.

Remember the beginning of your clinical work? It was difficult and you made mistakes. With practice things became easier. The same is true for research. You cannot wait until you are able to do a flawless piece of research, just as you could not postpone treating clients until you were expert at it. However, before you start to do research there are some tricks of the trade that make that first piece of work a little easier to do and a little better in quality, just as there were some techniques that you learned before seeing your first client. This book will give you some techniques for research.

Be aware that there is a psychopathology of research. The hunch, the original idea, is a uniquely personal thing, different from a psychotic delusion only in the sense that the research hunch can be tested in reality. Some people nourish these hunches so closely to their own hearts that their ideas are never allowed to see the light of day. They do this partly because they fear criticism from others, partly because they may be too critical of themselves. Excessive self-criticism and a need for perfection are often worse than no critical ability at all. Your first piece of research does not have to be a masterpiece. People put off starting to do research far more often because they may fear ridicule than because they fail to have ideas.

As we said above, there is great satisfaction in finishing a piece of research. It should be within the grasp of many more mental health workers than currently undertake research. The harvest is truly exciting, and the laborers are few, so — have a go!

Chapter 2

How Has
Mental Health Research
Been Done?

There are many methods and approaches to research, ranging from a simple anecdotal report to the most complex and counterbalanced design. The strategy to be used and the complexity of the questions to be asked in research depend on the current state of knowledge in the particular field to be investigated.

This chapter presents a description of various research strategies and designs. We hope that you will see it as a source from which you can gather ideas. There are many acceptable research strategies, each one appropriate to a different research endeavor, a different research hypothesis, a different state of knowledge in a given field. Here we simply present these strategies side by side. Subsequent chapters will help you select the most appropriate design for the research question that you pose.

Foulds and Bedford (1975) describe the various research strategies as follows:

> We will consider studies which make comparisons between groups, within groups, and within individuals. Each in turn may be handled cross-sectionally or longitudinally. This gives rise to six types of question, for which examples might be as follows:
>
> Between-group cross-sectional: "Are men more extroverted than women?" when the question is answered by

taking samples of men and women at one particular point in time.

Between-group longitudinal: "Is the decline in intelligence with age greater among men than among women?" when the question is answered by following up men and women over time.

Within-group cross-sectional: "Are depressives more X than Y?" when the question is answered by taking a sample of depressives at one particular point in time.

Within-group longitudinal: "How do depressive symptoms typically develop over time?" when the question is answered by measuring depressive symptoms repeatedly over time in a group of depressives.

Within-individual cross-sectional: "What psychiatric symptoms does Mr. X have?" when the question is answered by studying Mr. X on one occasion.

Within-individual longitudinal: "Which symptoms of Mr. X change most, and most quickly, without formal treatment?" when the question is answered by following Mr. X over a period of time.

These six types of questions can be divided into a multitude of subtypes, some of which incorporate features not included in Fould's classification and some of which mix several basic categories of question. In the following, we list a number of design issues related to Fould's categories:

Research without and with intervention. All of Fould's examples happen to carry no intervention. This is how one typically starts, observing what occurs naturally. However, at a later stage of knowledge one often builds interventions into research. By manipulating one variable and seeing what happens to the rest, one can get a feeling for cause-and-effect relationships. Such interventions are often experimentally produced: "What happens to depressives if we give them thyroid hormones?" At other times, we observe interventions in nature: "Compared with normal families, what happens to children whose parents divorce when the child is 3 or 4 years old?"

Qualitative vs. quantitative research. Most of us, especially beginners, are biased to feel that only quantitative methods are acceptable in real research, because only quantitative methods result in numbers that can be analyzed. For example, the question, "What is the effect of soothing music on free fatty acid levels in depressed women between the ages of 30 and 40?" is clearly seen as a real research study, even though the results may not be earthshaking. A subjective description of what these women feel when hearing soothing music may enhance our understanding of depression, but it may erroneously be seen as less real research. This is a sad commentary on the general understanding of research, and it is wrong.

Qualitative research, without generation of quantifiable measurements is often crucial at the beginning of a new field of inquiry or when parts of different fields are brought together in a new way. It deserves much more respect. Strauss and Hafez (1981) argue strongly for systematically developing clinical intuition, and they have developed research principles for this kind of work. Examples might be: "What are the most salient emotional experiences of nurses who counsel terminal cancer patients?" or "Can one describe the cognitive and emotional experiences of a terminal cancer patient during the first two months after being informed of the prognosis?" Frequent examples of qualitative research are anecdotal reports (e.g., "What are the staff and patients' experiences with a program of group counseling for cancer patients?") and phenomenological observations (e.g., "Being married to a successful professional woman"). They are often the only available research data in a new area.

Retrospective vs. prospective research. Research can be done by examining records of past events ("Do the deaths listed as suicides in New York City during the last five years have the same neighborhood distribution as population density?"). Retrospective work has the advantage that the data are already collected. A problem is that these data may be biased or the information you want most is incomplete or not available.

Prospective work is done by setting up an hypothesis, developing procedures to test this hypothesis, and then gathering new data to test the hypothesis ("Will four groups of depressive patients, matched for X and Y, show any differences in depression scores when a double-blind medication regime is carried on for four months?"). Prospective research has the advantage that we can plan what we want to study and are not biased in our predictions. The disadvantage is that we then have to spend long hours collecting the data.

Studies contrasting groups versus correlational studies. In group studies we contrast different *kinds* of things, seeing how groups differ from each other, e.g., unipolar versus bipolar depressives, or treatment with medication versus treatment with psychotherapy. In correlational studies we search for relationships between variables. Examples might be straight correlational studies ("Does the severity of depression in a certain group relate to the degree of overweight?") or the assessment of more complex relationships ("Does increase in height in dwarfs, undergoing X therapy, correlate with emotional readjustment as measured by the MMPI?"). Correlational studies also might involve studies of genetic variables, normative developmental observations, structural characteristics, or family characteristics ("Does the manifestation of recessive characteristic X covary with the tendency to affective disorder?"). Or they might relate present status with past behavior ("Among prison inmates convicted of crimes with various degrees of violence, what are the frequencies with which various forms of child abuse are represented?").

Which is the best of these strategies? It depends on the state of knowledge in a given field. If you think you have discovered a new disease, some anecdotal case reports will be exciting research. As we write this, a simple, uncontrolled case series of successful AIDS treatments would be superb research, if the cases and the treatment were well described. However, if you want to work on the effects of diazepam on generalized anxiety, you had better have a much more sophisticated design, addressing a question that has not previously been answered and replicated.

In sum, the more researched a given area is, the more sophisticated and well designed a new study has to be to contribute valuable new data. In areas where knowledge is lacking and little research has been done, much simpler designs are acceptable because even they add considerably to our knowledge.

Chapter 3

How to See Each Client
as an Experiment

An excellent way to start developing a research attitude is to develop systematic, testable hypotheses and ideas about specific clients. This chapter will show you one way this might be done.

One of the strategies that a beginning researcher can use to advantage is to select an interesting diagnostic category and then attempt to understand and treat a number of patients in that category with a questioning attitude. This will often lead to the publication of case reports (see Chapter 14) and to formal research on the topic later on. For example, you might be interested in clients over 65, in sex offenders, alcoholics under 30, self-mutilators, suicide attempters, or certain types of manic-depressives. Once you have determined your special group, a sensible way to go about the next step might be as follows:

(1) Find a recently published article that touches on some of the important points of your chosen diagnostic category. (2) Go to the individual in charge of computer searches at your library (see Chapter 6 on how to review the literature). This person will help you find key words under which the article was referenced and will do a computer search for you. (3) Read the literature uncovered by the search. (4) Develop a strategy for assessing and following clients.

In doing this work, first ask, "What do I think we know?" Then, "Do my patients feel or behave as we think they should?" Compare your experience with that of the published literature. If you see something different in your patients than you can find in the literature, if you are interested in this difference, and if you think it might be important, you may well be on your way to important research. Similarly, you are well on the way to a publishable study if the literature offers contradictory hypotheses about the phenomenon and your patients can either support or refute one of these hypotheses.

USING A FLOW DIAGRAM

In clinical practice (as well as in research), three of the most important steps are (1) gathering data and developing hypotheses (or vice versa); (2) arranging data and hypotheses into an integrated picture that describes the patient, the problems, and appropriate treatment procedures; and (3) communicating this formulation to others as a means of organizing the treatment of the whole patient.

A helpful organizing strategy for characterizing patients, developing an inquiring attitude, and measuring some central aspects of their behavior is spelled out in the following paragraphs. It involves a flow diagram. See whether you can follow this approach with a few of your own cases. We find it useful because it provides structure and forces us to speculate about cause-effect relationships in our patients, about treatments that might follow our hypotheses, and about ways to evaluate these treatments.

Our flow diagram is shown in Figure 3.1. Start with the column marked "Target Problems." List the various problems for which the patient is seeking help. Use the "Stimuli" column to list important historical events and possible causes or triggers that might set off these target problems. The "Presumed Internal Processes" column lists guesses (hypotheses) regarding internal (psychodynamic) variables that might link those stimuli to the target problems. The "Treatment Methods" column is used to list and sequence possible treatment procedures for each of the target problems, and the "Evaluation Methods" column is used to specify the procedures by which we try to monitor the patient's status so that the impact of our treatment methods can be determined. This last column is crucial in the development of a research attitude. Unless we develop ways to assess the effects of our interventions, we have no way of improving our approaches.

Name ————————— Education ———— ——— —— Marital Status — Referred by ·· ——— —— ——

Date ——————— Age———— —— Occupation ·· —— ———— ——— ··· Presenting Problem ————— · ——————— ··

Stimuli	Presumed Internal Processes	Target Problems	Treatment Methods	Evaluation Methods

FIGURE 3.1. Flow diagram format

Figure 3.2 shows an initial flow diagram drawn after the first intake interview. The patient was referred for bulimia. Notice how fast one gets a feeling for some factors that may drive this patient's bulimia. Notice also that already some systematic evaluation is planned for events surrounding her bulimia. You will see that two problems are little understood after the first hour: the patient's suicide attempt and her possible lack of social skills.

As treatment continues the flow diagram is updated whenever new ideas or data can be added. As it always does, the picture gradually becomes more complex for our patient (Figure 3.3). It developed that this patient was severely troubled by complex developmental and psychodynamic issues. The most important of these issues seems to be her relationship with her judgmental and controlling mother and a resulting complex of issues involving anger and control. Figure 3.3 shows our hypotheses about the relationships among these psychodynamic issues and between these issues and other problems. Notice that even this more complex flow diagram gives an easy overview of the salient issues. Take, for example, the column entitled "Treatment Methods." A team approach has evolved, with therapist C doing the behavioral work, coordinating it with an exercise coach and with those

doing medical and dietary work, while also referring the patient to another therapist for treatment of intrapsychic problems.
Our theoretical preferences also dictate the inclusion of a

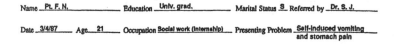

Name __Pt. F. N._____ Education __Univ. grad._____ Marital Status _S_ Referred by __Dr. S. J._____

Date __3/4/87__ Age__21__ Occupation __Social work (Internship)__ Presenting Problem __Self-Induced vomiting__
and stomach pain

Stimuli	Presumed Internal Processes	Target Problems	Treatment Methods	Evaluation Methods
Being alone Memories of first sex partner	Self theory: unattractive, fat, guilty, angry, depressed Punished enough, won't get fat	Overeats (feels full) Vomit Lack of social skills Suicide attempt	1. Continue assessment 2. Systematize food purchasing and eating 3. Systematize exercise	Record keeping of urges to eat beyond scheduled amount or outside scheduled times Miles and times (set up schedule for running) Do record keeping on best and worst social experience each day

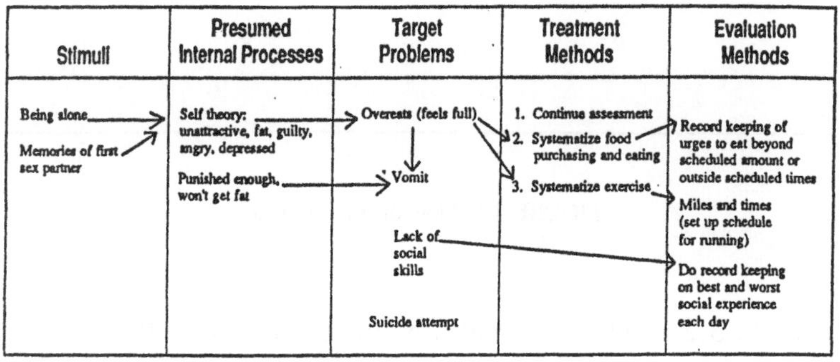

FIGURE 3.2. Preliminary flow diagram for a self-inducing vomiter

Name __Pt. F. N._____ Education __Univ. grad._____ Marital Status _S_ Referred by __Dr. S. J.__
Date __3/4/87__ Age__21__ Occupation __Social work (internship)__ Therapist _C_ Presenting Problem __Self-Induced vomiting__
and stomach pain

Stimuli	Presumed Internal Processes	Target Problems	Treatment Methods	Evaluation Methods
Being alone (not asked for a date) Social situations Memories of a series of enjoyable but secret and socially unacceptable sex experiences with a married man who has moved across the continent Vomiting discovered on 2/25/87 Mother interviewed (judgmental and controlling) Father interviewed (passive and aloof)	Self theory: "Large—I want to get fat; I'm not attractive to most men; I have sinned; I am soiled goods and probably unworthy of true love; I am a good runner and would like to run in marathons; I think I could be a good wife and mother." Anxiety Lonely, unloved; rejected because I am too fat; angry; afraid of losing control or being controlled. Tension "Guilty, Unworthy, soiled goods." After vomiting pt. feels less likely to get fat ("The calories are gone") and less uncomfortable and guilty ("Somehow the suffering of vomiting atones for my sins; I don't want anyone to know I've sinned or that I vomit.") Depression (Zung Index)	Overeating and self-induced vomiting 1. Pt. is alone usually on Friday or Saturday evening—urge to eat. 2. Purchases and eats large quantities of doughnuts, cake, bread 3. Feels full and uncomfortable (Feels "even more fat".) 4. Induces vomiting with finger ULCERS confirmed 3/1/87 Stomach pains: (for the last 6 mos.; intense in social situations) Social behavior: (seems agitated and hurt—avoids close relationships by being rude when she feels attracted to someone) Suicide attempt on 2/27/87	1. Systematize food purchasing and eating. 1. Daily exercise (marathon training with the club coach) in the late afternoon. 1. Medical management, dietary management (exercise has been approved) 2. Progressive relaxation 3. Biofeedback (SCL temp) for control of autonomic function 4. Social skills training 1. Individual psychotherapy by therapist D	Keep record of urges to eat beyond the scheduled amounts Keep daily records on weight, food purchases, eating, and exercising. Miles and times, refer to schedule set up by coach. Medical measurement in 3 mos. Use pain questionnaire for record keeping of stomach pain, frequency, and severity. Record PRN pain medication taken. Weekly esthus and daily record keeping of best and worst social experience. Weekly Zung Index.

FIGURE 3.3. Sample flow diagram

"Self-Theory" (self-image) section in the "Presumed Internal Processes" column. Under this label we include the patient's descriptions of her interests, strengths, weaknesses and other important characteristics. Often we indicate the sequence of the different treatments we are planning, estimate the number of sessions for each treatment procedure, and indicate the evaluation criteria that will determine whether a particular procedure should be continued beyond the estimated number of sessions. However, some of these details are omitted from Figure 3.3 in order to present the format with less clutter.

Another widely used road map for dealing with behavioral and emotional disorders is the ABC approach (where *A* stands for antecedents, *B* for behavior and *C* for consequences). This ABC approach to the understanding of patients is compatible with the flow diagram and can be used to develop separate initial descriptions for each of the problems presented by the patient. The ABC strategy can also be used in the initial interview and in preliminary communications with consultants and referring agents. However, the simple ABC diagram does not easily lend itself to a description of internal processes or to the matching of assessment and treatment procedures for the various problems. The obvious temporal sequence (flow) of the simple ABC diagram can easily be incorporated into the flow diagram format; the arrows in Figure 3.3 indicate some of our hypotheses about temporal sequences.

Finally, the flow diagram format facilitates communication with consultants and collaborators from outside the mental health professions. The various medical procedures of assessment and treatment are conveniently described and scheduled on the same page with the psychotropic medications and psychotherapy or behavioral therapy. We often use our flow diagram when we present clients to supervisors and to case conferences.

SUGGESTED STEPS IN ASSESSMENT AND DATA ORGANIZATION

Although the approach may vary among different mental health organizations, we have found that the research attitude of the established clinician is often fostered and supported by enlisting the client as a co-investigator. For example, at the end of the first session, most clients can be given a record-keeping assignment tailored to their presenting problem. At the very least, clients might be required to log the status of their presenting complaints once per day, between suppertime and bedtime. Or a phobic client might log the number of panic attacks three times per day, before each meal. For each panic attack, the client would note the situation and the severity of the panic on a scale from 1-5. (We have found that tying these observations to specific, routine behaviors such as eating increases the likelihood that the forms are filled out.) Alternatively, one might ask that only a description of the most anxiety-provoking experience of the day be logged. The record-keeping data sheet is then brought to each session and discussed. We have found it useful in the treatment of difficult kinds of clients, and it may also yield some initial data for research.

A problem often encountered when seeing each client as an experiment is the need to collect baseline data against which to judge therapeutic interventions. The clinical needs of the client often demand that treatment be started immediately, while the experimental needs require that we collect a nontreatment baseline, often lasting two to four weeks, before treatment can be started. In these situations, Houtler and Rosenberg's (1985) idea of a retrospective baseline has often been helpful. Basically, during a very early interview one collects as much information as possible concerning the variables in question during, say, the last four weeks (e.g., severity of symptoms, number of incidents of maladaptive behavior). This information is obtained as carefully as possible from the client and often from other sources: from significant others, from previously written critical incident reports, etc. At regular intervals throughout treatment, or at least at the end of treatment, one then obtains similar retrospective information, *using exactly the same procedures* as were employed during the collection of the retrospective baseline. While bias cannot be eliminated in this way, at least the data points are collected in the same way and are thus more or less compatible, while the client has been spared a possibly unethical delay in needed treatment.

Following one of the quantifying steps outlined here, most clinicians will naturally get drawn into the questioning, scientific attitude that is the beginning of all research. When the ratings given by a client don't follow logically from the events as we understand them, one is forced to rethink the formulation and consider alternate hypotheses. We believe that this procedure not only makes us better researchers, but better clinicians as well.

Chapter 4

Ethical Issues
in Mental Health Research

The pursuit of truth must be tempered by a realistic knowledge of social implications, as well as by an evaluation of what it will cost to get the desired research data, especially in terms of human cost.

This book is intended as a short, practical guide for the beginning mental health researcher. Unfortunately, we cannot discuss here all the philosophical issues of a scientist's moral obligation to pursue or not to pursue the truth in socially sensitive areas. That deserves a much more thorough exploration than we could give here. Suffice it to say that the desire to seek the truth and the imperative to respect individual rights and societal values often may pose moral dilemmas. Mental health workers should be guided by the tenets of the Nuremberg Code of 1946 and the Declaration of Helsinki, as published in the World Health Organization Chronicle, vol. 19, pp. 31-32, January, 1965 (see Appendixes 1 and 2). However, the issues are really much broader than those raised in these two documents.

There are many research activities that at one time would have seemed correct and legitimate that now would seem to be clearly unethical. For example, 20 years ago a medical student was involved in some research on uterine muscle. Every time there was a Cesarean section he would go to the operating room, and the surgeon would give him a little piece of uterine muscle. At that time this collection of little pieces was considered fine by everyone. Currently, such behavior would be considered highly unethical because informed consent was not obtained from each patient.

During recent years, most institutions have established guidelines and procedures to control the interaction between researchers and human subjects. However, even with these guidelines and procedures, daily research activity is usually an individual pursuit, and there is very little ongoing scrutiny by others. Thus there are continuing challenges to the researcher's integrity.

Besides the ethical issues involved in doing research on humans, there are many others, such as the ethical restraints of not plagiarizing ideas and quotations from other authors without appropriate acknowledgment, not suppressing data that do not fit the hypothesis, and not overstating the care with which the data were collected. It is surprising how difficult these issues sometimes are.

One of the greatest ethical challenges in research stems from the fact that good research activity can provide tangible rewards in terms of career advancement (publish or perish) and the esteem of colleagues. With such pressures on you, and often working totally alone, your integrity is often severely tested. Say, for example, that when completing the collection of 12 months' worth of data and doing a 3-month analysis of them, you find that mildly significant results can be made highly significant by ignoring the last three subjects that were collected. What a temptation. However, if the purpose of the scientific process is to advance knowledge and to provide information from which others can build, then each piece added to our knowledge should be solid. At least, if it is shaky, this should be clear from the report. It often takes the utmost integrity to honestly present marginal results. Nevertheless, in the long run it often pays, even if you lose a publication or two. Remember the last three subjects that were mentioned, the ones that changed a highly significant result obtained in 12 months' full-time work into a marginal one? This actually happened to one of us, 20 years ago, during the PhD thesis. Because of these last three subjects, the research conclusions had to be seriously qualified and were much less exciting and publishable. A nuisance then, but with 20 years' hindsight, a blessing. Based on subsequent research, the original conclusions (without the three subjects) would clearly have been in error, would have misled the field, and might have adversely followed the researcher for much of his career.

While these more factual research responsibilities are clear, there are many other dilemmas that arise in research activities involving humans. For example, if there are data to show that a treatment is effective, is it ever justified to withhold treatment from a given client in order to test whether, there is a placebo effect?

You are often not the best one to judge ethical issues in your work, because your focus on your research needs might bias your decision. To deal with ethical problems in human research, and to assure adherence to the internationally accepted guidelines of the Nuremberg Code and the Declaration of Helsinki (see Appendix), medical centers have developed research review committees or institutional review boards (IRBs). These committees and their composition are mandated by the Department of Health and Human Services (DHHS) if grants are supported by that department. These committees often include lawyers, oncologists, pharmacologists, internists, surgeons, psychiatrists, clergy, and institutional administrative officers. They could and should also include lay members of the community.

Once the IRB is approved, it is given wide authority to act on approval or disapproval of all studies performed by members of the institution. Operating within DHHS guidelines, the IRB is essentially a system of decentralized peer review on ethics. All research within an institution must be approved by the IRB if any DHHS research funds are received by that institution. In addition, no other federal agency will grant funds unless the investigator has received the institution's IRB approval.

Above all, the IRB serves to protect research volunteers by assuring conformity with ethical and legal requirements for consent. The committee examines the protocols for potential harm to the volunteers, both psychological and physical, and evaluates the necessity for the study. The IRB protects the investigator as well as the volunteer. You are legally and ethically much safer if your work has been examined and approved by the IRB.

THE ISSUE OF COMPETENCY

Recently the issue of the volunteer's, or client's competency to give informed consent has been raised in the case of psychiatric inpatients. Some of the DHHS's rulings imply that institutionalized psychiatric patients, as a group, may be incompetent to provide true informed consent. These rulings are responses to perceived past abuses involving psychiatric patients. Nevertheless, the concept of global incompetence of psychiatric inpatients is clearly difficult to defend. Ironically, it comes at a time when courts and society at large are judging that the vast majority of mental patients are indeed competent, as witnessed by the restoration to the institutionalized patient of previously denied rights, such as voting. Nevertheless, anyone planning to do research on institutionalized patients should be aware of this sensitive area and take especially careful steps in delineating for the IRB how the informed consent procedure will be conducted in such a case.

THE INFORMED CONSENT PROCEDURE

The ethical issue most pertinent to mental health research is the informed consent procedure. This is the aspect of a research project upon which the IRB focuses most intensely. The informed consent procedure is crucial because it is the means by which volunteers decide whether they want to participate in the study. They are told, in understandable language, what they are being asked to do, what the risks and benefits are to themselves and society, how or why they were selected, and how confidentiality will be maintained. The IRBs have taken the position that the informed consent should, in most circumstances, be written rather than oral. However, for projects where there is clearly no risk to the volunteer, oral consent may be permissible. When oral consent will be obtained, the investigator must submit in writing for the committee's review the exact wording of what will be said to the volunteer.

An informed consent document is easily written if the following seven points of the investigation are briefly addressed:

1. Title and purpose
2. Methodology
3. Risks and benefits
4. Permission to withdraw
5. Confidentiality
6. Investigator's name and how to reach him or her
7. Compensation statement

The language in a consent form must be clear and understandable to a layman, free of coercion, and easily read. The consent form should use the letterhead of the institution in which the investigator is based. A brief description of the project's purpose is important to give the volunteer an understanding of what the stakes are. The explanation of methods need not be detailed, but the volunteer must know if the project involves randomization to different treatment conditions and if it involves placebo or a nontreatment category. Also, the volunteer must know whether the investigation can be expected to be therapeutic, i.e., may be of personal benefit, or not. Volunteers must be told if alternative forms of therapy for their problem exist and what would be the risk of no therapy at all. In addition, all reasonable side effects and discomforts from medication or treatment must be listed. (The courts have ruled that reasonable means "what a reasonable person would want to know.") Further, the consent form should contain a statement assuring that the volunteer's present or future care will not be compromised for failure to agree to the investigation or for withdrawal from the experiment once it has begun.

The issue of confidentiality must be clearly addressed in the informed consent document. The common statement that "all information will be held in the strictest confidence" is insufficient. It is also frequently untrue. The volunteer should be told how the information gleaned from the research will be used, whether the individual participants in the research will be identified as such, or whether the data will be pooled without individual identification.

Another recent requirement of informed consent is a formal statement concerning financial and medical compensation in the event research results in physical injury. However, this statement can be omitted if the investigator and the IRB agree that the risk is minimal.

After the volunteer has read the form and asked all questions that occur, the consent form should then be signed by the researcher and by the volunteer. It is then dated and witnessed. If the volunteer is a minor, an adult must countersign the minor's signature. It is always wise to give the volunteer a copy of the signed document.

In sum, an adequate informed consent procedure clearly describes the investigation, neither states nor implies coercion, and gives the volunteers sufficient time and information to assimilate the full impact of what they are being asked to do. This is not merely a fulfillment of legal doctrine but also a requirement of good research. Failure to be clear in your goals can lead to skewed experimental results and even to erroneous conclusions. A clearly understandable explanation of the project to the volunteer does much to improve compliance. Thus, the informed consent doctrine, which initially might seem to be an unnecessary hindrance to research, may actually strengthen research design.

Chapter 5

How to Decide on an
Area for Research

Deciding on a research area begins with a few highly personal questions, such as, "Why did I choose a career in mental health?" or "What idea or case has really excited me in this field?" Once you have decided on a broad topic, this chapter will help you to make specific decisions about your own research focus.

Paradoxically, the practice of scientific research is largely an art. Like art, it can be a pastime or a profession, part-time or full-time, a refreshing and occasional counterpoint to one's major concerns or the dominant pursuit of a lifetime. Personal styles in research range from the compulsive drive of Michael Faraday, whose motto was "work, finish, publish," to the covert part-time perseverance of Copernicus, who gave final permission to publish his great work only on his deathbed.

Research is most exciting and meaningful when it grows out of questions or problems personally encountered in clinical work, rather than from an abstract decision to do some research. Often it will focus on phenomena that have puzzled you in doing clinical work. This kind of research has a high likelihood of developing into something you can call your own, and it can be carried out in close association with your clinical work. This will help in sustaining your motivation in the face of inevitable pitfalls and dry spells. We are recommending this sort of grass roots clinical research to beginners because it can give you a broad and intensive, first-hand exposure to what research is all about, from the excitement of recognizing a question you wish to examine, to the intellectual exercise of translating it into an experimental design with a workable methodology, to the sometimes tedious process of collecting and analyzing data, to the hard work of articulating your findings in written form for all to see and judge.

Before deciding on a specific area for research, an honest self-assessment should be attempted. Ask yourself, "Why do I want to do any research?" Is the effort based on your attempt to satisfy a requirement, impress someone, publish, or satisfy a long personal curiosity? The idea that research achievement is necessary for professional advancement initially should be given rather low weighting.

When you decide that you want to do research, there are two aspects central to your selection of an area. One is the personal factor, often unconscious or vague, which leads to specific interests and inspiration. The other aspect is the pragmatic factor of constraints within which you are able to conduct your work. Clearly the two are related, but for discussion purposes we will separate them.

The personal factor is easily explored by reviewing your past. What ideas, situations, or problems have stirred your interest and imagination in the field of human behavior? Was there a case, an article, a lecture, or an instructor that raised an idea you felt like pursuing further? Did you look up more information about some topic, or at least intend to do so? At this stage, even a far-fetched thought may be worth pursuing. Was there a related topic or research effort from your undergraduate, graduate, or medical school lectures in sociology, psychology, social work, biochemistry, physiology, neurology, or psychiatry you once thought would be fun to pursue? Consider the reasons why you chose a career in the field of human behavior. Let your imagination wander over past thoughts. Those thoughts can now be put into a much broader educational context, that is, a context extending from genetic and biochemical aspects to cognitive and affective aspects of family and social factors. In working with human behavior, feel free to consider other germane areas of knowledge such as anthropology, mathematics, jurisprudence, history, the arts, and philosophy. Few fields of study provide such a fertile area of research possibilities as does mental health.

After focusing on specific possibilities, try to find someone knowledgeable in that area, even if that person is in another department, in another school, or even in another town. Explore your interests, without feeling forced to reach premature closure on a precise question or hypothesis. Attempt to ferret out the current state of knowledge surrounding your ideas. Identify a few articles to review. Who are the respected researchers in the area? A few minutes of talking with a well established person in your area of interest could well save you many hours of library work and many false starts.

A personal fascination with some particular skill or type of gadgetry can both help or hinder research; in some cases it may be better kept as a hobby. Consider also the popularity of your area. Is it highly popular with colleagues? This may determine both the extent of competition and of excitement. Is it popular with society? This often largely determines the generosity with which the area is funded, as well as other derivative rewards and penalties. Of course, only the boldest and most competent should give a very low weighting to considerations of social and professional fashion, but those who completely capitulate to these pressures should perhaps not be in research at all.

Finally, in considering the personal factor, altruism or even a specific wish to help a particular patient may play a major role. This is quite all right. But also ask, "What is the importance of doing this research in terms of expanding the overall field of knowledge? What is its importance in terms of facilitating clinical work? Are there applications of this work in nonclinical areas?"

Having explored the personal factor, it is time to focus on the pragmatic factors by reviewing practical constraints. Available time, effort, and financial limitations are important considerations. Estimate the cost (in time and money) and possible funding sources. Can it be done less expensively by reconsidering alternate techniques? How much effort are you willing to put in? Assuming that you are busy now, what can you drop to make time for the research effort? As a general rule of thumb, we find that research projects typically take at least twice as long as we think they will take.

Ripeness of the area for significant discovery is another variable well worth considering. It may depend upon the development of new techniques, often from a different area or from a totally different discipline. Most budding investigators lack the experience to properly assess this factor, and outside advice may be helpful. In fact, a very good way to get involved in research is to select an investigator whose work you find stimulating. Indicate your interest in becoming involved in the research and then, under the investigator's guidance, assume some responsibility for a portion of it. While such projects have the disadvantage of not being entirely your own, this apprentice way of getting involved can provide useful initial research experience. It offers an opportunity for role modeling while working with an experienced investigator, it often is less fraught with trial-and-error learning, and it is more likely to yield publishable results, often with a substantially smaller investment of time and effort on the part of the beginning researcher than working it all alone.

Another important issue to be considered is your range of skills. They will limit your choice of a research area. They will also determine the nature and extent of collaboration and help that is required for success. Various forms of technical and statistical advice can be provided by consultants, and basic laboratory work is sometimes done by paid technicians. However, you should make sure that you are familiar with these procedures and techniques. A common fault we have observed in the inexperienced investigator is to assume that the abilities learned in graduate school or medical school are automatically sufficient in any area of research that is chosen, and that all other skills that might be required can be obtained by recruiting assistants or technicians. This subtle form of arrogance, we feel, is a major cause of much wasted effort and money in beginning research.

After you have settled on a broad area of investigation, you are now ready to hone it to a more narrowly defined target. Again, you will find that this process is a curious blend of personal idiosyncratic preferences and pragmatic constraints. The following list of questions may help to focus your work. It is not intended that this list be reviewed for conclusions at this point, but rather than it be used as a stimulus to help you move from the global to the specific. As you will see, the questions listed below are not exhaustive, there is overlap between them, and some of them are also discussed elsewhere in this book. Ask yourself:

1. Do you work best alone or in a team, supervised (like an apprentice) or unsupervised?
2. Are you going to do this in the clinic, a laboratory, the library, or at home? Is it going to involve humans (clients or nonclients), animals, or a review of records?
3. Is this going to be quantitative or qualitative research, group or individual, between or within subjects?
4. Is it going to be controlled or uncontrolled; not-blind, single-blind, or double-blind; retrospective or prospective; cross-sectional or longitudinal?
5. Are you going to look at predisposing or precipitating variables, or at variables that perpetuate the situation once initiated? Are there going to be interventions or manipulations, or are you simply going to observe what is going on?

Besides your own preferences, and the realistic situation you find yourself in, some of the answers to these questions will also depend on the state of knowledge in a given field and on what you want to get out of the research. For example, if you want to claim that A causes B, you will have to experimentally manipulate A and explore its effect on B. Even a well done longitudinal study observing the correlation between A and B over many years or decades will not let you conclude that A causes B.

As you think about these issues, the focus of your research will gradually emerge. As it does, you will be ready to do a preliminary search of the literature, as discussed in the next chapter.

Chapter 6

How to Review the Literature

A preliminary literature search can help to select an area for research, and it can help to formulate a research question. A more extensive literature search must then be done before final decisions on research design can be made. This chapter should help you become an efficient literature searcher.

Scientific and technical literature is much more thoroughly indexed than literature in other areas. Materials in psychology, education, and business are reasonably well indexed; unfortunately, material from the humanities is difficult to search thoroughly. A minimal amount of homework prior to instituting a systematic search pays dividends, and it is especially important prior to a computer search.

Begin by glancing at the printed edition of *Index Medicus* or *Psychological Abstracts*. Notice how it classifies and subdivides the topic area that you are interested in. This provides a good idea of the scope of the literature on a topic and may well assist you in further delineating your particular concern. There is a special section of review articles, by topic, which is worthy of attention. A recent edition of a standard textbook will usually provide general background information on the topic. Informal inquiries of your colleagues can also yield useful information and may even result in an opportunity to share a common research interest.

Once you have a grasp of how your area is classified, it is time to look for specific articles. In most libraries, data bases are now available for computer searching online. For example, the current MEDLINE file contains over 600,000 citations to journal articles listed in *Index Medicus* as published in the current and preceding two years. With the help of the reference librarian, a data base search can be completed in about 15 minutes. You have the option of printing the full record for each citation, including subject headings and the article abstract, or printing only the information necessary to locate the article, author, title, and publication. A retrospective search is also possible. The back files for MEDLINE extend to 1966. If a retrospective search is requested, the results will be mailed to your library in about a week. The cost of a data base search is minimal. A computer search generally yields more positive results than manual methods, since a computer can (a) handle several concepts simultaneously, (b) search an entire file and eliminate the need of looking in many index volumes, (c) retrieve items on new topics that might be hard to find through existing topic headings, and (d) isolate English-language publications or materials in any language.

This is not the point at which you will save time by sending a secretary or research assistant to do library work. If you do, you are likely to locate irrelevant references while missing important papers. Most reference librarians report that what users request and what they really want are rarely the same things. Make an appointment with the reference librarian and go in person. You can interact with the computer, and as you see what citations you are getting, you can exclude topics or redefine terms.

It should be noted that manual and computer searches will not necessarily yield the same materials. When searching the printed indices, you are limited to the controlled vocabulary and the limited combination of terms that the publisher provides. Only the title is used in determining these subject terms. However, when searching online, you can use common jargon, as well as the approved terms, by searching for the words and phrases not only in the title but in the abstract as well.

Current Contents, Social Science Citation Index, and *Science Citation Index* are worth special mention. *Current Contents,* published weekly, is essentially the tables of contents of scholarly journals. It is published in seven editions, three of which might be of special interest to you: *Clinical Practice, Life Sciences,* and *Social & Behavioral Sciences. Current Contents* is not the route to go in making a retrospective search because it is published weekly and does not have a cumulative index. It is an excellent way to keep current in your area of interest and build up your own reprint file. In a few minutes each week you can scan the table of contents of all the journals related to your interests that were published that week. Then choose the articles you would like to read and write directly to the author for a reprint. The addresses of the authors are listed in the back of each issue of *Current Contents*. Also, if money is no object, the publisher of *Current Contents* will send you copies of the articles of your choice as part of their original article tear sheet service.

The *Social Science Citation Index* and the *Science Citation Index* are based on the concept of citation indexing. Almost all scientific papers, reviews and correspondence refer to (cite) earlier papers that provide support or elaboration of the author's own ideas. In citing papers, the author identifies certain subject relationships. Thus a citation index identifies and groups together all recently published items that have cited the same earlier work. In effect, the earlier document becomes an indexing term useful in retrieving newer papers on the same subject. One of the major advantages of this approach is that it tends to overcome problems caused by changing and ambiguous scientific terminology. Both the *Social Science Citation Index* and *Science Citation Index* are available in printed volumes and online.

Although *Psychological Abstracts* (over 250,000 abstracts of journal articles in psychology from 1967), *Index Medicus*, or one of the citation indices is probably the best place to start, there are numerous other possible data bases, from *Foundation Grants* to *Pollution Abstracts*, including *Excerpta Medica* and *Biological Abstracts*. In addition, there are several other searchable data bases. For example, there is *Dissertation Abstracts International* — the entire file of theses, from 1861 to the present, in all subject fields (over 550,000 citations). The reference librarian is the person most likely to be familiar with these various data bases and can help you choose the most appropriate bibliographic tools.

If you have located a pivotal textbook or journal article, your search and your communication with the reference librarian can be greatly facilitated. Obviously the references cited in the pivotal article will be helpful, but other avenues are now open. For example, you can determine what key words your pivotal article has been indexed by and then use these key words to refine your search. You can also use a cumulative citation index to see what literature has cited your pivotal article since it was published.

Stacks, whether open or closed, and interlibrary loans provide the foundation for a wealth of information. Most items on the reviewer's list or printout can be retrieved easily and quickly from the stacks. However, an interlibrary loan (arranged through the Reference Department) takes time. A photocopy of a journal article will be provided generally within a week.

Condensing information into manageable proportions is a problem. Some items will be retrieved in book or volume form, only a fraction of which is pertinent. A photocopier, available in most libraries, can duplicate an entire item, the title page, or the summary. You may want to hand write a summary on 3 × 5 cards, or in a notebook. Take some time to organize these notes before you start writing so that you will not get swamped by them.

Categorizing and storing the collected information for later retrieval can be done in many ways. One of us has a system of photocopying only the interesting parts of an article or text, always including the first page with complete details about the source on it. These photocopies then are put into a set of large labeled envelopes or folders that stand alphabetized along a bookcase shelf. When an item should appear in several envelopes, it can easily be cross referenced by photocopying the first page as many times as necessary and noting on it the name of the file envelope where the whole item can be found.

As you gain experience with literature searching, condensing, categorizing, storing, and retrieval, you may develop your own favorite sources and methods. New systems, some computer based, are continually being developed, and we expect literature work to be easier for you than it was for us when we began.

Library work is like detective work, both exciting and frustrating. As you read and search, you will come across all sorts of tantalizing titles and tidbits to follow up. Many of them will be blind alleys. We know of no sure way to avoid them. All we can do is advise you to give yourself plenty of time and to document what you found where. Nothing is more frustrating than having to hunt down a reference you once read but now can no longer find.

Chapter 7

How to Decide on a Research Question

When you are formulating a precise research question, you are at a pivotal point in the development of good research. At this point in your work you collect all previous considerations, ideas, and guesses into one narrow focus: What do I want to know at the end of this piece of work? This chapter will clarify how to do this.

The quality and success of most research projects will largely be determined by a single phrase: the research question. Above all, it should be simple, understandable, answerable, and contain the very core of your study.

Up to this point, you have been dreaming about what you might like to do, playing with various ideas, checking the literature to see what others have done, and exploring what might be feasible. Now comes the time to make decisions, to commit yourself. You are at a pivotal stage in the development of your study. All previous considerations are now brought into one focal concept: the research question.

Consider again your chosen research area. Ask yourself, "What is it that I want to know?" If you cannot explain to yourself or to a friend what you want to know, then perhaps it is too early to decide on a research question. Restate your question in different ways until it captures the very core of your purpose. Now ask yourself, can such a question be answered? Would both your question and a possible answer be understandable to an intelligent layman? This often becomes an index of clear thinking.

It is axiomatic that success or failure in scientific research depends upon asking the right questions of nature at the right time.

This is often easier said than done. The problem is conveniently divided into two parts. The first depends upon the state of knowledge at the time the question is asked. The second depends upon technical considerations and the experimental situation in which you find yourself.

The state of knowledge at a given time plays a large role in determining the questions we are capable of asking. Good research asks a new question that has not been asked before, but a question that can be answered, given our current knowledge. Only the most imaginative can break totally out of the mold of current thinking, but it must be recognized that important research will always depend upon putting things together in a new light.

The research question is commonly expressed in terms of an hypothesis, which is an emerging theory or at least a piece of one. Since most scientific advances represent small steps, you are better to err on the side of modesty in formulating a question. Although a good question possesses an element of novelty, beware of the desire to ask the one crucial question that will result in the one pivotal answer. Although there sometimes are large breakthroughs in science, they are rare. Research more often proceeds in small steps. We all want our work to be relevant, unassailable, and crucial, but for your first few studies, modesty is also a virtue. Generally, it is better for the beginner to undertake a project that will provide the experience and satisfaction of carrying it through from the original idea to the final publication, rather than starting a larger project that does not get completed.

Besides the current state of knowledge, a good research question is guided by a variety of pragmatic factors. From your preliminary literature review and from your discussions with others, you already know what kinds of things are feasible to do, what kinds of methods are available, and what might be crucial variables that should be kept in mind. You also know what you can attempt in terms of effort and finances. These factors also determine your specific research question.

Let us imagine, for example, that you have read that an analogue of manic-depressive behavior has been observed in adult Chinese camels raised on plants that grow only in a certain part of China. Perhaps for your research question you would like to study Chinese camels, but if there are none around and no funds to go to China, it will be best to reformulate the question. Perhaps a similar behavior is seen in mice raised in the same parts of China? Importing mice might be more feasible. Or you might think about importing the dietary staples from China and raising your own mice on the Chinese diet. The question you then design will not be the original one, but one that moves in the desired direction and also is feasible. This far-fetched example is cited to help make a point: now is a very important time to think with great flexibility. The final research question will be different from the one you start out with.

Flexibility is also crucial when struggling with supposedly unmovable technical obstacles. To take a very simple example, consider the frequently used device of converting a very short amount of time into an easily observed measurement of distance. In this way, the progress of the very fast reaction between hemoglobin and oxygen was first observed by mixing the two reagents rapidly in a fast-flowing stream of fluid. The spectrum was then observed at different points along a tube. In a similar fashion, the complicated reactions of photosynthesis were first unraveled by mixing the reagents quickly and allowing the mixtures to drop from different heights into hot alcohol, which stopped the reaction. If the experimenters had attempted to measure the time variable directly, the research would have been either impossible or too costly in those days, because time could not be measured that exactly.

Once pragmatic concerns have forced you to reformulate your question, recycle the new one through the steps outlined earlier. Do the Chinese mice still hold the essence of your question, or were you, maybe unconsciously, after something else? Ask the old questions again: "Who would be interested in the findings, and why?" or "What might the clinical or theoretical payoff be?" or "Will the findings extend or clarify earlier research?" or "Will the findings raise new questions or open up new areas for investigation?"

Other ways that can sometimes sharpen the research question include attempting to express it in a few simple mathematical symbols or in a block diagram where the various concepts are connected by arrows implying direction and type of effect. This may seem inappropriate in mental health research, yet such exercises are often worthwhile because your concepts can sometimes be clarified and strengthened in this way. In suitable cases, the exercise leads to clearer exposition of significant variables involved in the hypothesis.

As your research question adjusts to personal, scientific, and pragmatic realities, you will find yourself going back to the literature a few times to see if the revised question is still relevant and to find out what has been published so far on the new angle that you have developed. What we are describing here is how a good research question gradually evolves and matures as you work with it.

However, there is a time to say enough. With all the above ideas in mind, now try to compose the final very simple research question. Try to state it as a strong, direct hypothesis. For example, the question "Does x occur in y clients, and if so, what does it mean?" might be rephrased into the statement, "I believe that x occurs in y clients, and to know that it does would be important because it would support z theory." Later on, you will learn that this statement will have to be rephrased into a null hypothesis for statistical reasons. Also, most likely it will need all kinds of careful qualifiers. For right now, however, a strong, direct statement is preferable.

Once the question is phrased and settled, keep it handy to guide you through the maze of work that follows. Look at the question in a few days. Is it still clear? If so, congratulations. Remember that great advances in science have often come from very simple questions. Some have been so simple that in retrospect they almost seemed self-evident, such as Fleming's research idea that stated that there must be something in the spoiled petri dishes that inhibited the expected growth of the bacteria. Obviously—but a great breakthrough, nevertheless.

Chapter 8

How to Match Research Design to the Research Question

Research designs change while knowledge accumulates in any given field. The more advanced our knowledge, the more sophisticated must be our design for a new study. The goal of a good design is to prevent as many alternate hypotheses as possible from explaining the results of the study. To this end, one attempts to eliminate from the study as many possibly contaminating variables as possible, either by using control groups, by matching variables across the groups, or by randomization.

The goal of all research is to explore phenomena that have not previously been described or evaluated and to investigate new relationships between these phenomena. Many think it is only research if the experimenter manipulates one variable and sees how it will influence another, e.g., how institutionalization influences schizophrenia, how a given drug influences the incidence of speech with paranoid content, how a specific type of therapy influences depressive behaviors. True, if you can predict successfully the outcome of such manipulations, before they are actually carried out, the goal of understanding that aspect of the phenomenon is at hand. However, most areas of mental health research are not yet at the step of manipulating a variable and predicting the outcome.

The approach you use in a particular research study will depend largely on the state of knowledge in that field. There seem to be three stages for the accumulation of new knowledge, each appropriate at a given state of development in the field.

STAGE 1: OBSERVING AND CATEGORIZING

You establish that a specific phenomenon does exist. You tally how often you can observe it, describe how it manifests itself, and clarify how it is different from other phenomena. Besides creativity, this requires a trained, open professional mind. You need to know where current knowledge still contains gaps. You need to notice if certain phenomena are unexpected, given the current state of understanding, but important enough to warrant scientific interest. You also need to observe very carefully, almost in an obsessive-compulsive way. Say you notice that a certain thought disturbance in one of your clients does not exactly fit into any of the currently available classifications. Describing how often it occurs and how it is different from other thought disturbances might be the beginning of an excellent research project.

STAGE 2: NOTICING ASSOCIATIONS

You explore various parameters of the phenomenon, or try to elucidate relationships between it and other variables. At this point data are gathered without manipulating the phenomenon; relationships are tallied by frequency counts or described by correlations. You are exploring how the new phenomenon fits into other parts of our knowledge. Hypotheses are then developed, based on these observed associations. For example, you might observe that the new thought disturbance that was recently described occurs mainly in young males who live in a certain community, that all but two of the people who are showing it are school dropouts, or that most are very religious, or that almost all come from a certain ethnic group. Comparing your observed associations with expected frequencies (chi squares or correlations), you will start to develop hypotheses about the newly discovered thought disorder. What else is similar among these patients? Could these other similarities explain their strange thoughts?

STAGE 3: MANIPULATING VARIABLES

Holding most variables constant, you now try to systematically vary one parameter that you consider important to evaluate the hypotheses that were developed in stage 2. If predictions that were made based on these hypotheses turn out to be correct, you gain confidence that you understand the new phenomenon. For example, if you feel that the new thought disturbance might be based on dietary insufficiencies because most of the people showing it seem to follow a strange diet, you may now start to vary diets or test whether other people, living in different areas but having a similar diet, might also show the new thought disorder.

The above discussion is placed here to emphasize that your research design, as well as the research question, will depend largely on the state of knowledge about the phenomenon. Entire scientific fields are sometimes working on stages 1 and 2, much as mental health did around Kraepelin's time when observation and classification were the main issues. Much of mental health research today is still at level 2. Smaller problems may be taken through all three stages by the same researcher.

It is often believed that true research only involves stage 3, the manipulation of variables. Actually, this is the only step that can occasionally be left to experienced technicians. To discover a new phenomenon and to generate hypotheses about its association with other events and variables needs a very creative, incisive, research-oriented, professional mind. It is often much more basic to research than to manipulate variables, as is done in stage 3. Working in stages 1 or 2 is something that the clinician is particularly well trained for, because clinicians have learned to be relatively unbiased and open minded in evaluating the phenomena that patients bring for treatment.

However, we will not be able to talk much further about stages 1 and 2. There are fewer teachable rules in these early stages, they depend heavily on intuition, a creative mind, and a thorough knowledge of the field in which you are working. For example, in the thought disturbance example described above, you could not have noticed the new and potentially exciting thought disturbance in your client unless you were open minded and knew a fair amount about many other types of cognitive dysfunctions that have already been documented.

For stage 3, the manipulating of variables, a certain universal set of procedures has developed. These procedures will be discussed in the rest of this chapter.

Suppose you hypothesize that a good program of psychodrama will decrease depressive behavior on an inpatient ward. Suppose you measure depressive behavior on a ward for three months, then train some staff members in psychodrama, have them do it on the ward, and then measure depressive behavior again for three months. Assume that you find less depressive behavior during the second three months. You would like to conclude that your hypothesis was correct, psychodrama does decrease depressive behavior. Such a conclusion is possible, but a number of alternative interpretations are equally plausible, even though they might be far less exciting. It is possible that something important outside of psychodrama occurred in the three months of the study. Maybe the staff grew more enthusiastic about their jobs, now that the researchers take a daily interest in them, and this affected the patients' depression. Further, seasonal differences in the incidence of depression might account for the difference in outcome. Or, if the clinical staff were aware of your research interest, in an unwitting attempt to please they might now put more emphasis on the well behavior of their patients. Suffice it to note that there are additional possible interpretations. This confounds the understanding of a possible relationship between psychodrama and depressive behavior. Despite your honest efforts and good intentions, little more will be known than before the experiment.

The principal concern in good research design is to eliminate possible alternative explanations of experimental outcomes. This is typically done by studying control groups, control individuals, or control times. *Controls* are groups, individuals, or times that are as equivalent as possible to the experimental ones except that they do not receive the active manipulations. A researcher tries to match experimental and control conditions, or experimental and control groups, on all pertinent variables except the one of interest, so that changes can be ascribed to it. In our hypothetical example, the experimental subjects with psychodrama and the control subjects without psychodrama should be matched on all pertinent variables except for psychodrama. This means that everything except psychodrama would have to be the same for both groups, for example, the time of year, other treatments they receive, the enthusiasm of the staff, the amount of time staff spends with patients, and the diagnosis of the patients. Most likely, this will not be possible, but the researcher approximates the idea as closely as possible.

The issue of adequate controls is complex. In the example above, more is changed than simply psychodrama if one group gets it and another does not. Staff morale may be better if they are trained in a new technique, if they receive added attention from the researcher, if they are more involved in patient treatment. On the other hand, less attention will be paid to other tasks if psychodrama is added to the other chores without adding personnel. To control for these confounding variables, one typically develops a credible placebo, i.e., another treatment for the control group that is similar in most aspects except for the active ingredient. For example, if it is the psychodrama that is crucial, the control ward might rehearse skits not related to the patients' problems and the staff might be told that trying to get into the role of somebody totally different was hypothesized to be therapeutic.

Obviously, adequate controls for an experiment involve many considerations. The major categories of concern are typically (1) the subject (2) the situation (3) the sequence of treatments, and (4) the experimenter. Each of these will be discussed.

SUBJECT-RELEVANT VARIABLES

Subject-relevant variables are any subject variables that might influence the outcome in a systematic manner. For example, sex differences have been demonstrated on a number of complex cognitive tasks. It obviously would pose major difficulties in evaluating an experiment in complex cognition if one group were largely composed of females and the other largely composed of males. While age and sex are often matched among groups because they affect so many things, what other variables have to be matched depends largely on the experiment. In a study on attitudes about abortion, religious beliefs might be an important variable to match or control, but in a study evaluating nerve velocity, the matching of subjects on religious attitudes would be ludicrous.

A second major category in this area is subject expectancies. In some cases, due to regulations regarding informed consent (see Chapter 4), it will be necessary to inform the subject of exactly what to anticipate. This procedure might influence subsequent performance. However, even if nothing at all were said or done, subjects would have their own preconceived ideas about the experiment and these, too, would influence performance. Equalizing expectancies is crucial in mental health research. Telling subjects that they will see a therapist soon while telling others that they have been placed on an indefinite waiting list will powerfully affect subsequent behavior over the next few weeks, even if nothing else is done.

SITUATION-RELEVANT VARIABLES

Any systematic difference between experimental situations could confound the interpretation of results. This is often a problem when groups from different mental health institutions are used for comparisons. More narrowly, if testing was done for one group in Room A and for a second group in Room B, group differences could be attributed to temperature or humidity differences if they differ between the two rooms, especially if the dependent variable is some kind of psychophysiological recording. Similarly, if you compare the efficacy of two biofeedback groups for the treatment of headaches, both groups might need to be run concurrently by the same staff. Over the course of the experiment, staff may become more efficient and experienced, but also less enthusiastic about their work, or the headaches may change with the seasons, and these factors may affect the outcome.

SEQUENCE VARIABLES

If a sequence of activities is involved in the experiment, interactive effects may account for some results. For instance, if you are interested in the effect of Drug A on motor performance, you might inject Drug A and then test your subjects first on Task 1 and then on Task 2. Assume you find that Task 1 is not affected by the drug, but Task 2 performance is impaired. Having put all your subjects through the same sequence, you do not know whether the poor performance on Task 2 is directly related to the drug, which might not have reached peak blood levels until Task 2, or whether fatigue or attention span might have changed over time and affected performance on Task 2. Counterbalancing often helps, i.e., giving Task 1 first in half the cases and second in the other half. Books on experimental design often feature very elaborate ways of counterbalancing, especially if more than two tasks are involved (look under Latin square or Graeco-Latin square designs).

EXPERIMENTER EFFECTS

Rosenthal (1966) has ably documented the subtle influences experimenters may exert on research outcomes. The danger of bias is particularly strong when technicians, students, or subjects, eager to please, are aware of the hypothesis to be tested. Ideally, the person actually interacting with the subject should be unaware of the hypothesis to be tested. The greater the blindness of both experimenter and subject, the less likely it is that the outcome will be contaminated by experimenter bias.

A second type of bias could arise when one experimenter is associated with one treatment, while a different one is associated with the second treatment. This is often done in psychotherapy research when different methods of doing therapy are to be contrasted. Obviously, in such a situation the observed effects could be attributed either to the different treatment approaches or to the different personalities of the therapists—a very difficult problem. Even when the same experimenter gives all treatments, he or she might still be differentially effective, consciously or unconsciously preferring one treatment method over the other. In an attempt to minimize such bias in a study assessing different schools of psychotherapy, you would probably need many therapists of different orientations, each doing all the different kinds of therapy. Obviously, this should tell you that there are research problems better not attempted by a novice.

Related to the above problem is the expert effect that has plagued many a researcher. This effect occurs when one technician has some magic that allows the reliable reproduction of a particular phenomenon. The expert effect is discovered when the technician resigns and the phenomenon cannot be reproduced. The lesson here obviously is not to allow any one experimenter to do everything, but rather to work in a team where more than one person can do each of the steps in the experiment.

Among other variables, the sex, status, and ethnic background of the experimenter have often influenced mental health research. Subjects bring certain expectations to the situation. Even if, for example, the female experimenter acts exactly like her male counterpart, she still might evoke different responses in her subjects. As a case in point, during the 1950s a number of researchers reported a phenomenon called *perceptual defenses*, in which subjects could not perceive sexually loaded words though correctly perceiving neutral words. The researchers interpreted this difference in perceptual threshold as defensively motivated. Interpretations changed when it was noticed that the effect could most reliably be produced when the subject was male, the researcher was female, and the words were "screw" and "tampon" (Postman et al., 1980).

CONTROL PROCEDURES

Controlling for many of the confounds that were discussed here can be accomplished mainly in two ways: matching and randomization. Matching means making sure that a given trait (e.g., age) is as equally distributed as possible among the different groups to be studied. The more traits you want to match, however, the larger a reserve of potential subjects you will need. Once matched on the most crucial variables, the rest of the potentially important variables are typically taken care of by scrupulous randomization. For example, if you want three groups of subjects for a given experiment, matched for age, sex, and social class, you would select from your subject pool triplets of people who are close to identical on these three variables. You would then randomly assign one member of each triplet to each of the three groups, hoping that this random assignment will equalize among the three groups the other variables that might be potentially important, such as intelligence or race. A further advantage of such randomization is the statistical fact that the amount of expected variability among the three groups can be reliably assessed and mathematically dealt with.

By now you may ask how you can possibly be aware of and deal with all these many potential confounds. You simplify the problem enormously if you are well versed in the pertinent literature (see Chapter 6), knowing which variables have already been shown to be important in previous research and which ones have been investigated and found to be irrelevant. This limits the number of parameters you need to attend to. Rarely, however, will you be able to control everything that still needs to be controlled. The perfect experiment has not yet been designed. In all research you ultimately have to strike a balance between what is ideally desirable to do and what is practically achievable. The answer to cost-efficiency questions will help make those decisions. How much will the knowledge to be gained from your experiments be improved by controlling a certain variable, and how much will it cost you in terms of money and time to control it?

Table 8.1 lists some relevant variables and methods for their control. This table, though cursory, does illustrate the fact that certain definite procedures are often employed to control particular confounding variables.

TABLE 8.1. Relevant variables and appropriate methods for their control

Relevant Variable	Control Procedure
Subject-Relevant Variables	
Demographic variables	Match groups on the most important variables[1] and randomly distribute uncontrollable variables
Expectancy	Blind[2] or equalize expectancies among the different groups
Situation-Relevant Variables	
Room, temperature, different institutions	Match groups on variable, or use the same situation alternately for members of the different groups

TABLE 8.1 (continued)

Attitudes and excitement created by the study	Develop believable placebo for the controls
Sequence-Relevant Variables	
Fatigue, learning, interactional effects	Balance order of treatment among groups [3]
Experimenter Effects	
Bias	Blind
Expert effect	Balance work among different experimenters
Sex, race	Match

[1] Matching. For each value of a variable in Group A, there is a corresponding value of the same variable in Group B.

[2] Blind. Experimenter and subject are unaware of the hypothesis for the experiment and the kind of manipulation used, and they do not know the expected outcome.

[3] Balance. The sequence of the treatment is different for each person in the group, making sure that each of the various treatments is given first, second, etc., an equal number of times and that each treatment follows each of the other treatments and equal number of times.

Chapter 9

How to Select the Variables to be Studied

Having decided what issues or concepts you want to study, you now need to find instruments to measure your observations. In mental health research, this frequently means selecting questionnaires and rating scales that must be valid, reliable, sensitive, and economical. This chapter shows how to assess these instruments, and cautions against developing new instruments too casually.

The selection of variables to be studied is crucial for any study. Variables must be selected for their ability to address the research question with accuracy and clarity. How one measures these variables is also important. Which scale you pick might well determine whether or not the study finds the hypothesized relationship, and this choice may doom your study even though the research thought may well have been correct. For example, if you want to measure the variable of hostility in dream reports, there are at least 15 scales in the literature that claim to do this! Unfortunately, these scales correlate very little with each other (Winget & Kramer, 1979). Obviously, not everybody agrees on what the term *hostility* means in dreams.

At the beginning of your research work, you usually start with a feeling for some relationships between concepts. Assume that you want to show that psychotherapy ameliorates neurotic behavior. Both of these concepts are very fluid. One person's psychotherapy is another person's supportive counseling. One person's neurotic behavior is another person's normal idiosyncrasy in the face of stress.

Most researchers advise that you first define the essential aspects of the phenomenon you wish to study, and second, determine the means for detecting and recording those aspects. This process, described in this chapter, seems rather arid, like textbook descriptions of the scientific method (of which Einstein was said to have remarked that, of course, it was nice, but one didn't really think that way). Before delineating the phenomenon formally, it can often be appropriate initially to play out in uncritical fantasy what you would like to find at the end of your research; there is time for careful analysis later.

Science depends on publicly observable and replicable phenomena. If your study is to be useful, other researchers need to be able to repeat it. This means that you have to carefully spell out what you mean by the concepts you use, and how you measure them. In our example above, once you spell out in detail how you plan to measure neurotic behavior, you have operationalized the concept for your study. Other researchers might not agree that what you measure is actually neurotic behavior, but they can understand what, in your research, is meant by this term and they can try to replicate your findings.

A common error when looking at research instruments is to assume that all measurements have to be done in absolute scores. Not so. Modern statistics can handle almost any relationship that involves some assessment of amount or size. For example, concerning the amount of psychotherapy in the above example, you might base your assessment on the following types of measurements (more of this in Chapter 10):

    a. "Yes" versus "no" (e.g., therapy versus no therapy). Easy as this sounds, it may be difficult to prove that your control group actually received no therapy, because you can hardly prevent them from seeking other help, or at least friendly attention, if nothing is forthcoming from you.

    b. "Little" versus "much." All patients might receive a certain minimal amount of therapy, but some might receive more, e.g., three times per week instead of once. This may be much more easily achieved than type (a).

    c. Rank ordering the amount of therapy. Instead of "little" and "much," you might increment the amount in smaller steps such as "minimal," "some," "much," "very much."

d. Measuring the absolute amount, e.g., hours of therapy per week. This might sound easy at first, but you will have to decide whether or not to measure only formal therapy, or whether informal contacts also have to be included, such as sympathetic discussions with other personnel on an inpatient ward. Also, there may be chitchat within the hour. Will you use only useful time? Simply assessing the hours that the therapist and patient spend together may not be what you want.

As one progresses from (a) to (d) types of measurements, scales become progressively more sensitive, i.e., they pick up more information. It is obvious that the less sensitive the instrument with which you measure the effect, the more cases you will need to assess the phenomenon and reach statistical significance.

TECHNICAL CONSIDERATIONS

Type of Instrument

Research in mental health spans a range of inquiry from chemistry to sociology. Consequently, mental health research uses a wide variety of instruments. On an informal continuum from the most to the least specialized, these instruments range from biological measurements through highly specialized performance tests, structured observational tallies, observational ratings and self-ratings, to open-ended interviews and self-reports. There are often trade-offs between the exact molecular precision of, say, a neuroendocrine assay, and the global inclusiveness of a general interview. Most mental health research uses instruments in the middle range: tests, rating scales, observations, and questionnaires. Any selection of measuring instruments in these areas usually requires weighing a complex set of factors.

Tests usually ask a subject to respond to a carefully structured set of stimuli, problems, or directions. For example, you might observe a child in a room with a given set of carefully selected toys. Such a standardized testing situation offers advantages in precision and control over less planned situations, but it also requires that the observers be competent and the subjects cooperative. Usually it does not escape the subjects' notice that they are being tested. This may change their behavior. Paper and pencil tests are used more often than behavioral observations because they require fewer resources. However, behavioral tests, such as asking the subject to cooperate with a colleague of the tester in accomplishing certain tasks, may better measure the real-life phenomenon you are trying to study.

Observer rating scales can often be completed by a paraprofessional. They can be inexpensive and unobtrusive, but the variations in interpreting the meaning of the scale items can be distressingly wide. Using untrained observers, this results in more error in the assessment than one would like to have. Scale items must be defined as clearly as possible. For example, it may be better to require a tallying of very narrowly defined social behaviors, rather than asking for an overall rating of social competence.

Self-administered scales and questionnaires require more competence and cooperation by the subject than observer ratings. They also involve risks of idiosyncratic interpretation of the test language by the subject, but their advantages in economy and in direct contact with the subject without intermediaries lead to their frequent use for subjects who are not seriously disabled. Self-administration does not, of course, limit the data to subjective measures ("How strongly do you feel . . . ?"). Subjects can be asked to report on objective measures as well ("How many times before noon did you . . . ?"). Under the proper circumstances, well motivated subjects can be expected to keep surprisingly accurate records of events.

Structural Considerations

Validity is the most serious question faced in the selection of a measuring instrument. Does the instrument in question actually measure what you want to have measured? Remember, the real variable to be studied is the real-life phenomenon that the researcher believes to exist and wants to assess. Under the operational assumption that the instrument captures the essential characteristics of that original phenomenon, the measures obtained by the instrument actually become the phenomenon to be assessed, at least for the duration of the study. You will not be working with depression, for example, but with check marks on a questionnaire that represents your operational definition of depression.

Validity in mental health research is difficult to establish. There are no Standard Units of Depression or Schizophrenia. It may help to discuss three types of validity:

Face validity means the obvious relationships of the scale items with the phenomenon to be studied. If you study depression, asking whether a person feels "blue and sad" or "suicidal" has more face validity than asking whether the person feels constipated.

Empirical validity involves previous research indicating that the question to be asked does actually relate to the underlying phenomenon. Asking whether a person has insomnia when you want to know whether the subject is depressed has more empirical than face validity. There is no obvious reason (on the face of it) why insomnia should relate to psychiatric depression, but empirical (research) evidence has shown that the two are related.

Construct validity is the most difficult but also the most important to assess. Does the scale actually measure the essence of the construct (e.g., depression) that it says it measures? Remember the 15 dream scales that assess hostility, each in a different way? Which of these scales measures the kind of hostility that you are interested in? No one study can give you the answer to construct validity. You need to evaluate many studies and to see how the scale in question behaves in each of them. A scale labeled *depressive index* is probably not measuring the construct we call depression if it consistently disagrees with clinical judgment or if it consistently finds more depression in males than in females.

Ultimately, construct validity in mental health research often rests on expert consensus. Any major variable to be studied in your work should be assessed by well established instruments that possess adequate construct validity. However brilliant your work in other aspects, if other researchers cannot relate your findings formally to work whose validity is unquestioned, they may ignore it. On the other hand, including some scales with less established validity, say for following up a weak hunch, occasionally reaps unexpected rewards. Now and then researchers temporarily lay aside their announced research question in order to publish more exciting serendipitous findings obtained by these more marginal scales.

Reliability is much easier to measure and can be a partial indicator of validity; it is a necessary but not a sufficient condition for validity. Reliability is the extent to which the instrument produces the same scores when the measurement is repeated under supposedly equivalent conditions. If two trained expert raters cannot produce fairly close agreement between them when scoring the same phenomenon, they do not have a reliable measure. Similarly, if on a supposedly stable trait measure such as "ego strength" your subjects score high one day and low on another, your measuring instrument for ego strength is probably not reliable (or it might not be valid, i.e., not measure what we mean by ego strength).

Two elements are important in developing reliable measures. If your measure involves clinical judgment, training is crucial so that the same observation or behavior gets the same rating each time. Different raters must assign the same meaning to scale items. Both general orientation and special training in the use of the rating instrument must be similar if an instrument calling for clinical judgment by a rater is to be reliable. The other necessary element to improve reliability is a careful definition of the task. No amount of training can make up for a task that is too broadly defined. This was found, for example, in the development of a depression scale. Well trained psychiatrists achieved only low agreement when they tried to classify whether a patient was depressed. However, their reliability improved considerably when they were asked to rate the intensity of the patient's depression (Beck et al., 1961). Similarly, rating how much a person has improved tends to yield quite low inter-rater reliabilities. There are just too many sources of variance that can affect such a score. Breaking the task into separate ratings for before and after treatment may produce more reliable improvement scores.

Sensitivity is another issue when selecting measuring instruments. How fine a gradation can the scale assess reliably? For example, if you wished to demonstrate that a particular intervention was effective in raising performance on some scale by three units, but the scale was normally accurate only to within two units, demonstrating any effect would be next to impossible. One instrument may simply be more sensitive than another, or it may depend too heavily on the type of rater. These phenomena are well illustrated in a comparative study of the sensitivity of various rating scales to various drug treatments (Raskin & Crook, 1976).

The range of an instrument indicates the population for which it was targeted. This range is closely related to sensitivity. An instrument developed for the purpose of delineating distinctions within a specific group may not differentiate effectively outside that group. The Minnesota Multiphasic Personality Inventory (MMPI), developed to help in diagnosing psychiatric patients, will not differentiate well among the different personality traits that occur within the normal range. On the other hand, the California Personality Inventory (CPI), developed for assessing normal personality dimensions, would be a poor instrument for clinical diagnosis. Different populations may need different tests. This may even be true within the same personality dimension. A depression scale designed for use on a psychiatric inpatient ward may not be suitable to assess minor fluctuations in depressive moods that occur in normals.

PRACTICAL CONSIDERATIONS

Cost and Subject Involvement

The costs of your scales, both for staff and clients, need to be weighed against benefits when choosing assessment instruments. These costs are not all economic. For example, if other staff or clients with limited commitment to the research are involved, asking too much of their time will pose a threat to the integrity of the data. Questionnaires may be filled out carelessly, or less motivated clients may drop out, thus leaving a biased sample.

There are several things you can do to keep such losses and inaccuracies to a minimum. You can make sure that the research protocol does not call for skills or judgments that are beyond those who are asked to respond. You can increase involvement by keeping people as informed or involved in their tasks as the design will permit. You can try to minimize the paperwork, make the tasks easier or more interesting, say, by use of a computer display, or you may synchronize data collection with preestablished routines. In the absence of carefully controlled studies on these factors, however, it is hard to know how much good they do.

The involvement of human subjects has direct implications for validity. When people participate knowledgeably in research, they do so not only as subjects (which really means as objects for examination) but also as observers of their participation. Their reactions as observers may in some cases threaten the validity of the findings. It is sometimes worthwhile to use unobtrusive measures, in which the possibility of a subject play acting is ruled out. In other instances, an unobtrusive measure might be used as a control variable, to demonstrate that subjects' reactivity to being tested was not significantly distorting their performance. Clearly, the use of these unobtrusive variables may not extend to a violation of the requirements for informed consent.

Developing Your Own Scales

Researchers often face the important issue of whether to use or adapt existing instruments or whether to develop, from scratch, an entirely new instrument or assessment device, e.g., a new questionnaire. A custom-built scale may seem more attractive because it would assess exactly what you are looking for, but it may be relatively time consuming and difficult to develop because issues of reliability and validity need to be settled first. Nevertheless, the huge library of tests and scales in psychology is testimony to the perennial researchers' conviction that they can build better instruments, rather than borrow old ones. However, the vast majority of instruments so developed have seen little use, and the research done on them is lost because it does not tie into existing bodies of knowledge.

Economy of effort is, of course, only one of the reasons for using old instruments. The community of scholars is limited in time and energy needed to accept new measures. You need to demonstrate that the new measure significantly improves the old ones. This may require carefully assessing and understanding the limitations of the old scale before offering a new one. If the old scales have been used in many research projects, tying into that network of relationships with your new findings may far outweigh the advantage of having a newly developed scale, even if the new one is objectively better. At the very least, you should be quite convinced that existing instruments are entirely inadequate before starting a new one.

Nonetheless, it is inevitable that at some point most researchers become involved in at least modifying a scale. If that is all, you may not have to become involved too deeply in the techniques of scale construction, because the incorporated elements for the old scale can serve as comparative references validating the new. Beyond that stage, however, you should begin by exploring both theory and examples of the art involved in developing new instruments. See Nunnaly (1978) for theory and Hamilton (1967), or Beck et al. (1961) for careful comparisons among alternative depression scales as an example of what may be involved. Overall, it is a difficult and time-consuming endeavor to develop a new questionnaire or scale. Resist the impulse, unless a new scale is truly needed and you have the required time to develop it.

Selecting a Scale

With all the theoretical considerations discussed so far, how does anyone ever get to the point of selecting a scale? Happily, the procedure is not as complicated as the theory suggests.

If you work on a problem that is similar to one addressed previously by other researchers, start by evaluating the scales and measurements that were successful in the earlier studies. Initially, select from the scales they have used. Narrow the number of possible instruments to a very few. Don't be afraid to write to the authors of the earlier research. Ask them for their reasons for choosing a particular scale. The goal of publishing papers is to disseminate information, and your inquiry indicates to the authors that this goal has been achieved. Most will be only too happy to discuss their work with you. Or call the authors if writing did not get you anywhere; some are too busy to reply by letter but may be willing to talk for a few minutes over the phone.

If your work is in a new and previously unpublished area, or if you truly cannot find any appropriate scales, look through the references listed below. If there is a good scale in the area of interest to you that has been used for a few years, one of these books should have a reference to it.

Buros. *Tests in print*. 1974.

This is an encyclopedic work concerning tests of personality, aptitude and achievement. It contains reviews and bibliographies.

Hargreaves et al. *Resource materials for community mental health education*. 1977.

This is an NIMH-published collection. Chapter 22 includes a review and examples of instruments oriented to program and treatment outcome evaluation.

Millon and Diesenhaus. *Research methods in psychopathology*. 1972.

This book contains a description of various assessment techniques in mental health research.

Raskin and Crook. *Sensitivity of rating scales completed by psychiatrists, nurses, and patients to antidepressant drug effects*. 1976.

This publication permits evaluating the appropriateness of scales to diagnostic, treatment, and personnel categories.

Research and Education Association. *Handbook of Psychiatric Rating Scales*. New York: Research and Education Association, 1981.

This is an NIMH-sponsored publication that reviews about 50 scales to diagnostic, treatment, and personal categories.

Sweetland and Keyser. *Tests*. Kansas City, Test Corporation of America, 1983.

This is a catalog of tests with a strongly educational and business orientation.

Winget and Kramer. 1979. *Dimensions of dreams*.

This publication lists most rating scales that have been used in the content analysis of dreams and other veral material. Discusses research pertinent to each scale.

Chapter 10

Frequently Used Assessment Devices

In this chapter we survey some frequently used tests and other assessment devices. We describe their background and uses, give an example of each, and list a source where the test or more information about it can be found. The list of devices we review in this chapter does not imply that these are the best or even the most used ones. We simply picked some of our favorites to get you started.

In the last chapter we discussed how to select tests and assessment devices for your research. The better a given test measures what you are interested in, the more likely it is that you can engage in a valid test of your hypothesis.

There are literally thousands of tests, questionnaires and other assessment devices. Each research area and each researcher has favorites. Some tests are used more widely than others, sometimes from sheer habit, sometimes because they are truly better than others.

In the following paragraphs we discuss some of the tests that we like and have used. This list of tests should not imply that these are the best tests. We are simply trying to get you started on your own list. If you are not currently searching for an assessment device, you might want to skip this chapter and save it for a later time.

In the following, we first outline two structured diagnostic interviews. Next we present four frequently used devices that require considerable training to administer and interpret. Unless you have had such training, you will need an experienced co-investigator who has used them. Finally, we have selected a few of the shorter paper-and-pencil assessment devices that require less training to use. For each of the devices that we discuss, we have described its use, given a sample and some background, and indicated a source where the test or some information about it can be found.

Before you use any of these assessment devices, you should know what was written by the original author(s) and later by authors who used or critiqued it. Locate these references through the Cumulative Citation Index or a computer search.

STRUCTURED DIAGNOSTIC INTERVIEWS

There was a time when the reputation or credentials of a professional alone was enough to validate a given diagnosis for research. No longer. Nowadays it is difficult to publish research using diagnostic categories unless you carefully specify the process by which you arrived at the diagnoses. This is most easily done using a structured diagnostic interview. You and your reader are then sure that you have asked all the important questions. Also, you will have all the diagnostic answers systematically collected should they later become important to the research.

Both diagnostic schedules discussed here start with a brief, relatively unstructured interview to get background information and clarify the essential features of the psychiatric problem, "letting patients tell it as they see it." The second part of the interview consists of specific questions that are usually asked verbatim.

The Schedule for Affective Disorders and Schizophrenia (SADS)

Description and Uses   This is a structured clinical interview leading to the diagnosis of many psychiatric disorders by research diagnostic criteria (RDC). The interview emphasizes depression and schizophrenia, but it also diagnoses many other psychiatric disturbances, anxiety disorders, substance abuse, and antisocial personality disorder because they need to be ruled out for a diagnosis of either depression or schizophrenia.

Sample

(Assessing social functioning):
"During the past five years, when was the period you had the most to do with other people socially?", then: "How much did you have to do socially with friends or with other people then?" (leading to a rating of 0-7, with definitions for each scale point).

Background

Leading up to DSM-III, there were research diagnostic criteria (RDC) for many psychiatric disorders. These criteria started with the Renard Hospital Group in St. Louis and were then expanded by a group at the NIMH Clinical Research Branch under the leadership of Spitzer, Endicott, and Robins. Although the NIMH project focused primarily on the depressive disorders, the ubiquity of depressive symptoms in other psychiatric disorders required the development of criteria for noneffective illnesses as well. The full version of the SADS has two parts. The first one focuses on current psychopathology; the second focuses on events over a lifetime. The full version takes two to three hours to administer. A shortened version, the SADS-L, is almost identical to the second part of the full SADS, and takes about one and a half hours to complete. Researchers often use the SADS-L because it does not assume that the patient is currently ill.

Source

Dr. Jean Endicott
Department of Research Assessment and
  Training
New York State Psychiatric Institute
722 West 168th Street
New York, NY 10032

Endicott, J. and Spitzer, R. L. A diagnostic interview. *Archives of General Psychiatry* 35; 837-844, 1978.

The Structured Clinical Interview for DSM-III (SCID)

Description and Uses
This is a clinical interview schedule leading to a DSM-III diagnosis. It simply lists, in a logical sequence, all questions that have to be asked to arrive at a valid diagnosis. It takes about one to two hours to finish, as does the SADS.

Sample
(Assessing past major depressive episodes): "Have you ever had a time when you felt depressed or down or had no interest in things for two weeks or more? . . . (if yes): Has there been more than one time? . . . When was the worst time? . . . Now I am going to ask you about that time. . . . Was there any change in your appetite?"

Background
Once DSM III had appeared, a standard format need to be developed to ask all the pertinent questions systematically, in order to make a diagnosis. The SCID is that standard format.

For each diagnostic category, the SCID first asks two or three screening questions. If the answers are negative, you can skip all the other details. Even so, the SCID is long and many clinicians ask only a part of it, e.g., all questions pertaining to anxiety or to depression.

Source
Dr. Robert L. Spitzer and Dr. Janet B.W. Williams
Biometrics Research Department
New York State Psychiatric Institute
722 West 168th Street
New York, NY 10032

ASSESSMENT DEVICES
THAT NEED CONSIDERABLE TRAINING

There are many assessment devices that require some training to administer, score, and interpret. Some of the most widely used are presented in a recent book by Newmark (1985). Four of these devices are briefly described in the following paragraphs.

The Minnesota Multiphasic Personality Inventory (MMPI)

Description and Uses

This is a 556-item, paper-and-pencil test with true or false answers. The MMPI evaluates certain dimensions of psychopathology, aids in diagnosis, and has been helpful in research on psychopathology.

Sample

"I often have strange experiences."
"Someone has control over my mind."
"I have never told a lie."

Background

The test was empirically developed by presenting more than a thousand items to a large group of normals and to individuals who had been previously identified as falling into one of eight diagnostic categories (including schizophrenia, paranoia, and depression). Through a series of analyses items were then selected that differentiated (a) between each clinical group and the group of normals, and (b) among the various clinical groups. In the present form of the test, there are ten clinical scales: eight syndrome labels and one scale each on masculinity-femininity and on social introversion. There are also four validity scales that are designed to detect major test-taking strategies or attitudes.

MMPI interpretation has matured over the years. One now diagnoses by profile, taking all scales into account simultaneously. This means that one no longer diagnoses, say, schizophrenia from a high schizophrenia scale, or depression from a high score on the depression scale. The highest two to four scales are typically the most critical for diagnosis.

Over the years, many additional scales have been developed on the 550 items of the MMPI. See Dahlstrom, Welsh, and Dahlstrom (1975) for a listing. Some of these new scales were done a priori, i.e., somebody simply selected those items that on the face of it seemed to be pertinent (e.g., Taylor Manifest Anxiety Scale). Others were empirically devised, i.e., somebody gave the test to two groups with different known characteristics and selected those items that differentiated the two groups.

Source

University of Minnesota Press
2037 University Avenue, S.E.
Minneapolis, MN 55414

Graham, J.R. *The MMPI: A Practical Guide.* New York: Oxford University Press, 1977.

The Rorschach Test

Description and Uses

This is the famous inkblot test. It employs ten inkblots that subjects are asked to interpret, describing what they see. This test was published in 1921 as a personality test. It is claimed that the Rorschach taps more covert (unconscious) processes than most other tests, partially because the subject does not know what the tester is looking for. Uses of the Rorschach now include, among others, an evaluation of personality dynamics, the monitoring of progress in treatment, and even identification of suicidal patients.

Sample

Inkblots are symmetrical about the vertical axis. One is often seen as a butterfly.

Background

Rival systems for scoring answers to this test have been a source of confusion since its inception. We like the Exner system to analyze the Rorschach. It seems that Exner and his colleagues have combined the best aspects of earlier systems and have developed a comprehensive and powerful strategy (Exner & Weiner, 1982).

There are two stages to the administration of the Rorschach. First the client is asked, "What might this be?" After responses to all ten blots have been obtained, the clinician and the patient go over each blot again to determine both the location of each response on the ink blot as well as the various aspects of the blot (e.g., form, color) that were influential in creating the response. From these data the clinician then codes the client's responses in accord with various stylistic features such as use of form, white space, color, and detail. Various scores are then calculated from these codes, and the clinician compares them to the norms for nonpsychiatric controls and for various clinical populations.

An assortment of interpretations can then be made. For example, the number of times the client uses only the shape of a blot to create a perception is compared to norms for both nonpsychiatric controls (who use shape as an exclusive determinant about 45 percent of the time) and for various clinical groups. To illustrate, it has been observed that schizophrenics use less pure form responses during acute episodes than during periods of remission. Similarly, use of pure form near the normative level is interpreted as indicating that the client functions in a relatively emotion-free or rational mode. Use of less form suggests that it is difficult for the client to perform in an affect-free manner. On the other hand, use of much more than the normative levels of pure form suggests that the client has too strict a control over affect and rarely allows affect to influence behavior.

Source

Publisher: Hans Huber, Bern, Switzerland.

Distributed by:
Grune & Stratton, Inc.
111 Fifth Avenue
New York, NY 10003

See also: Exner, J.E. and Weiner, I.B. *The Rorschach: A Comprehensive System*. New York: John Wiley & Sons, 1982.

The Thematic Apperception Test (TAT)

Description and Uses

The TAT consists of 31 black and white pictures, each mounted on a separate card. The client is typically shown a subset of them. Murray, the developer of the test, suggested 20 cards at two sittings, but other procedures are common. Some cards are more appropriate for adults, others for children. Some are suggested for males, others for females. Earlier cards in the series represent more realistic events; later cards show more atypical situations. No scoring system has achieved sufficient consensus to be recommended. The goal is simply to get the client's fantasy material and to compare it with stories that are typically told about the same pictures by normals. Murray then recommends an analysis of the client's needs and environmental presses.

Sample

In the first card a young boy is looking at a violin. The boy is often seen as concerned or emotionally aroused. The picture suggests that there may be an issue of achievement or motivation.

Background

This test was developed in the 1930s by Henry Murray. The stimuli of the TAT are far less ambiguous than those of the Rorschach.

The interpretation of the test can take many forms. Dana (Newmark, 1985) explains that initially the mechanical steps include a synopsis of each story as it stems from the particular card stimulus. There is subsequent cross-referencing for similar themes, conflicts, persons, settings, etc. Frequencies of occurrence and the particular cards in which they occur are noted. Finally, one interprets relative emphasis, importance, or personalization of thematic contents. Each TAT analyst has developed a set of interpretive guidelines, usually implicit, that can be applied to the summarized story data.

Among the more helpful guidelines or questions are the following: (1) How well do the stories correspond to the pictures? (2) How well did the client follow directions: is there a description of feelings, was an outcome described? (3) Did the test taker distance himself or herself from the negative feelings or behaviors described in the stories? For example, were the less acceptable behaviors attributed to characters who are like the client, or who are different from the client (e.g., sex, age, status, etc.)? (4) How literal are the stories with regard to the client's life and feelings?

Source

Harvard University Press
79 Garden Street
Cambridge, MA 02138

The Wechsler Adult Intelligence Scale — Revised (WAIS-R)

Description and Uses

This test consists of 11 separate subtests that take from 45 to 75 minutes to administer. The subtests are divided into categories of verbal intelligence (6 tests) and performance intelligence (5 tests). The administration and scoring are highly standardized.

Sample

Because the WAIS-R is so highly standardized, reliable, multifaceted, and widely used, we have decided to go into more detail than we have on the previous tests. Examples of each subtest follow:

(a) *The Information Subtest* consists of 29 questions about factual information. One of these asks, "Who was Louis Armstrong?"

(b) *The Picture Completion Subtest* consists of a series of 20 pictures, each with an important part missing. One of these is a picture of a frog with a leg missing.

(c) *The Digit Span Subtest* comprises two tasks. The first is to listen to the examiner say a series of numbers and then repeat the series. The second task is to listen to a series of numbers and then reverse the series and repeat it backwards. The digits-forward subtest begins with a series of three and goes to a nine-number series. Two trials are given at each length. "Digits backward" starts with a series of two and proceeds to eight. The testing continues until both trials at one length are failed.

(d) *The Picture Arrangement Subtest* consists of ten sets of cards with pictures. The client is asked to arrange the cards so that a story is told by the sequence. One of the sets consists of three cards that should be arranged to tell the story of a worker building a house.

(e) *The Vocabulary Subtest* consists of 35

words for which the client is asked to give a meaning. One of the words is "fabric."

(f) *The Block Design Subtest* consists of a set of blocks with which the subject is asked to copy a picture. There are nine pictures. The blocks are identical plastic cubes, red on two sides, white on two sides, and diagonally divided into red and white triangles on two sides. One of the designs is composed of four blocks and looks like this:

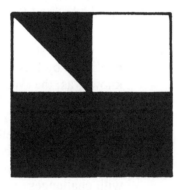

(g) *The Arithmetic Subtest* is composed of 14 math problems that are presented orally and are to be solved without paper and pencil. One of the problems asks, "If you have 18 dollars and spend 7 dollars and 50 cents, how much will you have left?"

(h) *The Object Assembly Subtest* presents four cardboard puzzles of common objects; the client is asked to assemble them as quickly as possible. One of the objects is a hand that is cut into seven pieces. (This subtest is similar to the Hooper Test of Visual Organization, described in the later section on brief tests and scales.)

(i) *The Comprehension Subtest* consists of 16 questions requiring the client to provide explanations. Some ask what the client would do in a hypothetical situation. One asks, "What should you do if while in the movies you are the first person to see smoke and fire?"

(j) *The Digit Symbol Subtest* involves a specific symbol for each digit from one to nine. The client must draw as fast as possible the appropriate symbols (e.g., a triangle) in blank boxes beneath a series of digits.

(k) *The Similarities Subtest* requires the client to tell how 14 pairs of nouns are alike. One pair is *dog* and *lion*.

Background   The general strategy of the WAIS-R was first published by David Wechsler in 1939 and was known as the Wechsler-Bellevue. This test was revised to the WAIS in 1955 and to the WAIS-R in 1981. The test reflects Wechsler's description of intelligence as a multifaceted and multidetermined global capacity that enables an individual to comprehend and deal with challenges.

The WAIS and WAIS-R have many uses, including vocational and educational guidance and neuropsychological evaluation. There are similar tests for children: the WISC-R for ages 6-16 and the WPPSI for ages 4 to 6-1/2. It typically takes about one hour to administer the children's versions, slightly longer for the adult version.

TESTS THAT REQUIRE LESS TRAINING TO USE

Hundreds of available assessment devices require little or no training to administer and score. We have selected a few for presentation here. Most of them would be best used with the advice or collaboration of a psychologist.

The Dartmouth Pain Questionnaire

Description and Uses	This is a five-part, paper-and-pencil questionnaire that enlarges on the McGill Pain Questionnaire. It is used to assess pain and its influence on various aspects of the client's life.
Sample	Part 1 is two outline drawings of a human figure on which the client indicates the location of pain. Part 2 is a list of descriptive adjectives from which the client selects ones that describe the quality of pain. Part 3 is a self-esteem assessment device. Part 4 is a record of pain severity during a 24-hour period, and Part 5 samples some fundamental pain behaviors as well as some of the remaining healthy behaviors (e.g., How much time in the last 24 hours did you spend lying down—awake? How much time in the last 24 hours did you spend out of your house?).
Background	This questionnaire evaluates both impairment and remaining function. Results indicate that remaining function is an important source of variance that can be particularly helpful in the selection of treatment and in the evaluation of outcomes.
Source	Corson, J.A. and Schneider, M.J. The Dartmouth Pain Questionnaire: An adjunct to the McGill Pain Questionnaire. *Pain* 19:59-69, 1984.

The Quick Test of Intelligence (QT)

Description and Uses	This is a picture-based, 50-item test of verbal intelligence. The client views four pictures and indicates which of them best depicts the meaning of a word. The examiner progresses through a list of words with increasing difficulty until the client misses six consecutive

words. The Quick Test can be used for a very rapid (5-10 minute) estimation of intelligence.

Sample

Four line drawings are shown to the client, e.g., one contains a scene of an automobile race and another contains a picture of a policeman controlling traffic. Two of the words are "contest" and "authority."

Background

This test can be used with a wide range of clients (from two years old and up; from retarded to highly intelligent). It provides a quick and approximate indicator of verbal intelligence.

Source

Psychological Test Specialists
Box 9229
Missoula, MT 59807

The Memory for Designs Test

Description and Uses

This is a 15-item test of memory for geometric line drawings. The test evaluates a form of spatial memory and perceptual-motor coordination. It can be used as a quick screening device for organic impairment and is often used to help differentiate between functional and organic impairment.

Sample

The subject is shown a picture of a triangle for five seconds and is then asked to draw the triangle from memory.

Background

The scoring strategy attends to various aspects of figure reproduction. Norms are available. Work habits and general attitudes can often be clearly observed during this test.

Source

Psychological Test Specialists
Box 9229
Missoula, MT 59807

The Hooper Test of Visual Organization

Description and Uses

This is a 30-item, picture-based test of ability to recognize simple objects that have been cut into several parts and rearranged. The Hooper test can be used to differentiate maturational from functional problems. The test has also been used to evaluate right hemisphere pathology.

Sample

The subject is shown a picture (line drawing) of a bench in five pieces and is asked to name the object that has been cut up.

Background

The scoring is simple, with 2 points assigned for correct identification, 1 assigned for near misses (listed on the scoring sheet), and 0 for a total miss. The client's responses to this test can provide clues about a wide variety of issues, ranging from test-taking attitudes to thought disorders.

Source

Brandywine Associates
P.O. Box 1
Concordville, PA 19331

Self-Rating Depression Scale (SDS), Also Called Zung Depression Scale

Description and Uses

This is a 20-item, paper-and-pencil test that is used to determine the intensity of symptoms of depression.

Sample

One of the items is "Morning is when I feel the best." The client selects one of the following answers: "none or a little of the time," "some of the time," "a good part of the time," "most or all of the time."

Background

This test is one of the most frequently used short tests of depression. It simply asks the client to note common symptoms of depression on a 4-point scale, and norms are provided for the total score.

Source

Merrell-National Laboratories
Division of Richardson-Merrell, Inc.
2110 East Galbraith Road
Cincinnati, OH 45215

Fear Survey Schedule (FSS)

Description and Uses

This is a 108-item test used to determine what specific stimuli or situations cause the client to be afraid. It is helpful in developing a complete picture of the fears that are bothering the client and in planning behavior therapy.

Sample

The client rates the various fears that are listed. How much disturbance would they cause? The 5-point rating scale extends from "not at all disturbed" to "very much disturbed." Some of the stimulus items are "being alone," "nude men," "criticism," and "loud voices."

Background

This test can be scored for general fearfulness, and some publications have provided data on large samples. However, it is usually used to evaluate fearfulness in specific situations so that appropriate treatment can be designed and the impact of treatment can be monitored.

Source

Educational and Industrial Testing Supplies
P.O. Box 7234
San Diego, CA 92107

Jenkins Activity Survey (JAS)

Description and Uses

This is a 52-item, paper-and-pencil questionnaire that evaluates the degree to which the client can be called "Type A" or "coronary prone." It has been used in both research and clinical settings and can be helpful in planning an individualized rehabilitation program.

Sample

"When you are under pressure or stress, what do you usually do?

1. Do something about it immediately.
2. Plan carefully before taking action."

Background

This questionnaire evaluates the client's tendency to be competitive, impatient, concerned about time pressures, and overly involved in professional or work issues. The JAS is well standardized and has been used in many published studies.

Source

The Psychological Corporation
c/o Harcourt Brace Jovanovich, Inc.
7500 Old Oak Boulevard
Cleveland, OH 44130

Rotter Internal-External Scale (IE)

Description and Uses

This is a 29-item test that evaluates the extent to which the client feels personal responsibility for events in his or her life. The test has been used in research and clinical settings and has led to a proliferation of other tests and to some important theoretical advances. It (and some derivative tests) have also been used as an aid in planning individualized therapy.

Sample

"Which do you strongly believe (pick one of the pair):

Many of the unhappy things in people's lives are partly due to bad luck.
People's misfortunes result from the mistakes they make."

Background

A forced-choice format is used, and the test yields a score that can be compared with several large samples. Rotter has provided a sample of 1000 adults.

Specialized versions of this testing strategy have been developed. One of these is the Health Locus of Control Scale (HLOC), which examines locus of control with regard to health and illness (e.g., ''I am directly responsible for my health.''). Wallston et al. (1976) have published this 11-item test.

Source   J. Rotter, *Psychological Monographs*, 80, 1966.

Wallston et al. *Journal of Consulting and Clinical Psychology*, 44, 1976—for Health Locus of Control Test, pp. 580-585.

Chapter 11

How to Carry Through
Your Research Project

Most research projects go through a pilot phase in which
the researcher fine tunes the project and makes sure it can be
carried out as planned. Then the researcher begins the main
data collection phase in a single-minded and determined
way, not deviating from the project unless absolutely necessary.

There is a large leap from the armchair planning you have
done so far to the actual carrying out of the project. If your project involves new procedures, scales that you have not tested yet,
or patients and settings that are not absolutely familiar to you, it
seems best to run the planned procedures on a few patients and
observe whether the results you are collecting make sense. This
is called piloting the study, and it typically involves a fair amount
of fine tuning such as changing procedures, studying patient
flow, writing out practically every part of the instructions, designing detailed data sheets and log books. It seems worth noting
that some of this work will have occurred during the selection of
the research question, and certainly before the presentation of the
protocol to the IRB.

Once this phase is over it is time for labor and determination.
Once you have started the main study, stick with your plan. The
time to redesign the study is over; resist the temptation to add
some new features. However, if you do come to some true im-
passe or some unforeseen severe complications, you might need
adjustments to keep the study going in the right direction. In that

case, remember your basic research question and decide accordingly.

The main problem for clinicians doing research is time. We have found it impossible to do research work unless we religiously set aside a block of time that cannot be infringed upon. If you wait until you can find time to do research, you will be 65 before you start. There is always some more clinical work that you could do for your clients, and they need it done today, while it always appears that research can wait. Well, it cannot. If it is important to you to do this work, it deserves a regular, scheduled time.

Label every piece of data that you collect, every sheet of paper, every observation, even though it is obvious to you during the collection phase what you are doing. Keep a log book of what you did every day. One of us (PH) once worked in a lab where a carefully designed study on the behavior of chickens was carried out. Over 200 animals were each put on various drugs in a carefully counterbalanced order, and they then were put through complex learning paradigms. The entire procedure was filmed carefully for later behavioral analysis. After two years of work by various technicians and graduate students, an entire room had been filled with films and data sheets. Then it was discovered that the labels on some film cans had not stuck well enough and that, for other films, labeling was incomplete. For example, it might be missing such information as what drug the animal had been on or even which animal it was. The log book had only sporadically been kept. For over half the films there was no way of reliably identifying which film went with what drug in what sequence. Over $50,000 and two years of an entire lab's work were lost. Therefore, label, and then label everything again. When the time comes to analyze, you will be grateful that you know exactly how each piece fits.

While you keep your mind on your study and doggedly follow the procedures outlined during planning, also keep your mind open for unexpected events. They are the germs of new studies and new ideas. Remember Fleming. He did not enter the lab planning to discover penicillin. He was engaged in another study when his petri dishes spoiled.

And keep the data clean. Assume you work all day with a

volunteer in a difficult vigilance study, tracking his alertness from morning to evening by giving him numerous vigilance tasks throughout the day. On the way out he tells you casually, "By the way, that was tough. I had a lousy night's sleep last night, and by 3 AM I took some sleeping pills which made me a little groggy today." Throw that data out, even though the volunteer might reassure you that he didn't think it affected his work today. Better to have no data at all than to have dirty data. Contaminated data confuses the issues, leads to erroneous conclusions, and prevents you or somebody else from studying the issue in a correct way. Remember, we are building knowledge that is supposed to last forever.

Chapter 12

How to Analyze Your Results

Statistics are used to make statements about large populations after measuring only a small sample of that population. The goal of this chapter is to teach you some statistical language and thinking so that you can knowledgeably discuss your research data with a statistician.

If you have never studied statistics, never had a course in the analysis of empirical results, you can learn this topic in one of two ways: You can either take formal courses in this field, or you can go through informal on-the-job training. Most mental health workers take the latter route. It simply means that you discuss your research project with somebody who is knowledgeable in this field and gradually absorb statistical know-how by doing actual work in this area.

Overall, the former route (i.e., a formal course) is preferable, but few have enough time to follow it. If you choose the second route, you need some basic concepts. Unfortunately, like most other specialists, statisticians have developed their own jargon and their unique methods of thinking, not immediately clear to the novice. This chapter gives you some of the background and the language needed to understand what a statistician is talking about. It will not teach how to actually do statistical tests, but with the help of modern computers, that is the least of your worries. Any technician or computer programmer can load your data into the computer and analyze it, once you describe what kind of data you have or what test to use. What you need is to know the basic concepts.

THE BASIC PROBLEM

Assume that you want to know how the depressed clients you are currently treating compare in age with the schizophrenics under your care. Simple! You ask each patient's age and compute the average, say 31.25 years for your schizophrenic clients, 52.5 years for your depressed clients (see Figure 12.1). Absolutely no statistical theory is involved here! You know for certain that, among the patients you are currently treating, your depressed patients are, on the average, about 20 years older than your schizophrenics.

Unfortunately, you are rarely interested in learning such simple facts. Rather, you typically want to extrapolate from what you know, generalizing from a small sample to some overriding truth. Do the above numbers mean, for example, that depressives in general are older than schizophrenics? How sure could you be that in a batch of patients that you treat in the future your depressives would again be older than your schizophrenics?

Statistics are used when you want to speculate beyond the sample that you have actually measured. In other words, statistics are used when you want to make statements about other samples that you have not yet measured, or about all people in a certain population. In the above sample, the rules of statistical inference provide guidelines to indicate whether any differences you observed between your two samples of patients (the schizophrenics and the depressives) are simply chance variations or whether these differences are likely to be observed repeatedly if new samples are randomly drawn from the same populations.

```
                                    Mean for schizophrenics
                                    | 31.25 years
  0 = schizophrenic                 |              Mean for depressives
                                    |              | 52.5 years
  X = depressed                     |              |
                                    0              X
                                    |    X         |   0
                      0      0    0 |    X     0   |   X
  Number of Patients  0      0    X |    X     0   |   X      X      X

  Age in Decades   0      1      2      3      4      5      6      7      8
```

FIGURE 12.1. Comparison of age of schizophrenic and depressed clients

LEVELS OF MEASUREMENT

Statistics deal with numbers. However, these numbers may have different levels of meaning. Before selecting appropriate statistics, you need to know the levels of measurements that you are dealing with in a given experiment.

Nominal numbers are symbols for categories or names, just like the numbers on football jerseys. Assigning number 1 to depressives, number 2 to schizophrenics, and number 3 to patients who show neither illness, we can organize the patients into groups. However, these numbers do not stand for amounts; they do not mean that two depressives are equal to one schizophrenic.

Ordinal numbers imply a relationship of more or less, say, more disturbed, less disturbed. Assigning a 2 to a more disturbed and a 1 to a less disturbed person gives us an ordinal scale.

Rank-ordering your data from most to least or from highest to lowest results in ordinal scales. Military ranks might form such a scale: say, general = 5, captain = 4, sergeant = 3, corporal = 2, private = 1. The distance between the ranks may be uneven without harming the ordinal scale, as long as the numbers are in the correct order.

Most rating scales used in psychiatry are ordinal scales. One often ranks on 5- or 7-point scales, say from "strongly agree" to "mildly agree," to "neutral," "mildly disagree," and "strongly disagree." Though the ranks are in proper order, you cannot assume a priori that the distances between the individual scale points are necessarily equal.

While it is often done, it makes no sense to add, subtract, or average ordinal data. The mean of two privates and one captain certainly does not equal a sergeant. Nevertheless, there are statistical tests that deal with ordinal scales quite well.

Interval scales have all the characteristics of ordinal scales, plus the requirement that distances between the various scale points must be equal. Intelligence quotients are assumed to have interval scaling, although there is reason for debate on this. If the IQ measures truly have interval scaling, this means that an improvement of 5 IQ points covers the same distance, whether a person improves from an IQ of 70 to 75 or from an IQ of 105 to 110. While it makes sense to compute averages or to add or subtract scores on an interval scale, multiplications are nonsensical when using interval scales. In other words, it makes sense to talk about an average IQ in a certain group, but a person with an IQ of 120 is not twice as intelligent as a person with an IQ of 60, nor three times as intelligent as a person with an IQ of 40.

Ratio scales give the highest-level measurements. In addition to equal intervals between numbers, ratio scales have a true zero. Multiplications make sense. Age is such a scale. A person aged 12 is twice as old as a person aged 6, three times as old as a person aged 4.

Ratio scales are rare in mental health research. Holmes and Rahe (1968) claim that their life stress units are ratio scales. Not only would this mean that the value for different life stresses can be added, but also that multiplications are allowed. If the Holmes and Rahe units really have ratio scaling, somebody with 300 life stress units per year could be said to be twice as stressed as somebody with 150 life stress units. Not surprisingly, Holmes and Rahe's claim of ratio scaling for life stresses has led to vigorous argument.

Knowing the level of your measurements is crucial in selecting appropriate tests. Siegel (1956) gives a thorough explanation of levels and other issues briefly discussed here.

CONTINUOUS VERSUS DISCONTINUOUS DATA

If you count how many, you are dealing with discontinuous data. You ask, for example, how many of your patients are male or female. There is no in between in such data.

If you measure some characteristic that can gradually change along a given scale, you are dealing with continuous data. Examples would be intelligence, aggression, age, income. Rather than asking how many clients are in each category, you ask how much of this quality each client has. Classifying eye color into five different categories is collecting discontinuous data; measuring pupil size gives you continuous data.

Sometimes, for conceptual ease, we create discontinuous data out of continuous ones. We may, for example, call all our patients either "bright" or "not bright" even though we know that intelligence is a continuous variable. Or we may classify patients into either "depressed" or "schizophrenic" or "other," even though we know that in real life these supposedly discontinuous groups gradually shade into each other.

DESCRIPTIVE PARAMETERS

To gain an overview of your data, you must summarize it. For discontinuous data, this typically gives you numbers per category (frequencies), e.g., 20 males, 18 females. Continuous data are typically summarized by two numbers: central tendency and variability (scatter).

The best measure of *central tendency* is the average (mean). However, means make sense only for interval or ratio scales. Another measure of central tendency is the median, i.e., the score of the person who is in the middle of the distribution if all scores are rank-ordered from lowest to highest. Another measure of central tendency is the mode, i.e., the score that was most often obtained. The median and the mode are appropriately used with ordinal data, where the mean does not make any sense.

Measures of *variability* (scatter) also depend on the level of measurement. For ordinal scales, the range is often given (highest and lowest scores in the group). Another commonly used measure of variability in ordinal scales is the quartiles, i.e., the scores of the individuals of the 25th and the 75th percentile. For interval and ratio scales, the standard deviation is usually given. This is a measure of how much the data cluster around the mean in a normal curve, an issue that we shall take up next.

The Normal Distribution

Many variables of interest to mental health researchers are said to be normally distributed. The scores of such a variable cluster around the mean in a symmetrical, bell-shaped fashion. In mathematical terms, however, not all bell-shaped curves are normal. Rather, the curvature of the bell has to follow certain rigidly defined principles, although the widths and heights of the normal curves can differ (see Figure 12.2).

Why should variables such as intelligence or height be nor-

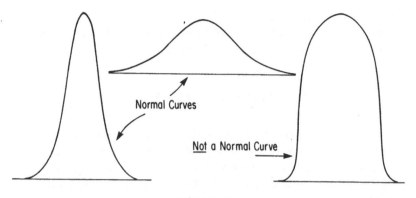

FIGURE 12.2

mally distributed? Whenever a variable is the sum of many independent subvariables, it is likely that the variable is normally distributed. The idea is that each of these subvariables can contribute either a positive or a negative amount to the total, independent of what others have already contributed. The sum of these subvariables, then, makes up the variable in question, e.g., intelligence or height.

Most individuals will cluster close to the mean in such a variable, because for most individuals some subvariables will contribute positive amounts, others negative. The overall population will contain very few individuals in whom almost all subvariables contribute positive amounts and very few individuals where almost all factors are negative. This is why most of us are near to average in intelligence. There are few geniuses and about equally few idiots. In other words, intelligence is normally distributed because it depends on many independent parameters such as genetic factors, early infant environment, nutrition, schooling, etc. For most of us, some of these factors were positive, others were negative.

Since most human traits are multidetermined, most can be assumed to be normally distributed in the general population. For example, most of us have an average amount of anger, self-esteem, or circulating growth hormones. Examples of traits that are not normally distributed are color blindness or the number of hallucinations that are experienced in a lifetime. In this latter example, most people would score only one or no hallucinations, while progressively fewer would range from 1 upwards.

One advantage of normal distributions is that they can be characterized by two numbers: Mean and standard deviation. For example, knowing that the mean IQ as measured by our intelligence tests is about 100 and the standard deviation is about 16 tells you much about the distribution of intelligence in our population if you know the normal curve (see Figure 12.3). For example, it tells you how many mildly retarded individuals you can expect (more than 2 standard deviations below the mean, i.e., IQ of less than 68), or how many geniuses (more than 3 standard deviations above the mean) you should have in a certain population. The larger a sample, the closer its mean and standard deviation approximate that of the population. Thus, the number of retardates or geniuses to be expected can be estimated more exactly in a large group such as a nation; there can be serious error if you talk about groups of only a few hundred people.

Figure 12.3 illustrates the area relationships of a normal distribution. Note that the greatest area, i.e., the greatest percentage

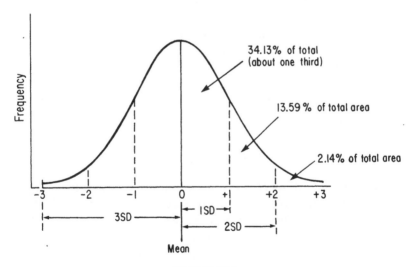

FIGURE 12.3.

of cases (about two thirds) occur within $+/-1$ standard deviation (SD) from the mean. As you move away from the mean, the area under the curve, i.e., the number of cases, decreases. About 95 percent of all cases lie within 2 SD).

THE NULL HYPOTHESIS

The following is a logical and an empirical fact: You can only prove that two things are different. You cannot prove that they are the same. Take the length of two sticks. If one measures 3 feet 2 inches and the other 3 feet 3 inches, you know for certain that they are unequal in length. If both measure 3 feet 2 inches, however, you have not proven that they are absolutely equal in length. Maybe under a microscope you could find that one stick still is slightly longer than the other. And if they were equal even under a light microscope, are you sure that they would be equal if you were to look with an electron microscope?

Because of the empirical fact that you can never prove equivalence but only difference, you always start with the assumption that the things you are comparing are actually equal. Let us return to the example of schizophrenics and depressives graphed in Figure 12.1. For that example, the null hypothesis requires that you initially assume that depressed patients and schizophrenics, on average, are the same age. With statistics you can then attempt to refute this null hypothesis. If you cannot refute it, you have not proven that the two populations are truly equal in age. You can, however, indicate that they are very similar, and with statistics, you can give a range outside of which the differences are unlikely to lie.

PROBABILITIES

Attempting to draw conclusions about large populations (e.g., all schizophrenics versus all depressives) from your small sample, you can never be absolutely certain that you are right. Even if you have used all the safeguards of good experimental design described in the previous chapters, you still might, just by pure chance, have found an atypical sample, e.g., a group of abnormally young schizophrenics. Thus, when you make statements about differences that apply to the general population on the basis of measuring a sample of the population, you are always dealing with uncertainty, with probabilities.

How large do the differences have to be before you can reject the null hypothesis with reasonable confidence? Assume that you are plotting the age of your schizophrenics and your depressed patients in that original sample (Figure 12.1). Note that although there is a sizable mean difference of about two decades in age between the two groups, there is also a great deal of overlap in the distributions of the two samples. The range of scores for each sample is rather great; you are seeing schizophrenics, for example, who are in the second and in the sixth decade of their life. These two observations, the amount of overlap and the two large ranges, suggest informally that the mean difference found here might not be significant.

The major point to be gleaned from this sample is the fact that the significance of a result is a function not only of the mean difference, but also of the variance (scatter) of the data. Large mean differences are relatively meaningless in the context of a large variance.

The role of many statistical tests is to provide a formalized way of weighing the mean differences versus the variances in a given experiment. Comparing mean differences between groups with the variances, statistical tests can then provide decision rules for determining whether the results of an experiment are reliable or whether they occurred by chance.

In an attempt to avoid personal bias, most scientists set a probability or confidence level before they start research. This is called p. Usually p is set as either .05 or .01. If you decide, for example, that you will require a p = .05 significance level, you decide that before you believe your findings, chances must be at least 19 in 20 that the differences you have found in your research are reliable, not generated by random error. Another way of saying this is that with a p = .05 you would, by chance, see a difference as large as you found in your experiment only once in 20 samples drawn from populations in which there is really no difference. If you set a significance level of .01, you specify that the chances have to be at least 99 in 100 that the differences you have found are indicating real differences in the population before you reject the null hypothesis. Obviously, how certain you need to be before you assume a real difference depends, to a large extent, on the gravity that may be attached to your findings. If you were testing for the toxic effects of some drug on humans, you might want to set a confidence level of $p = .001$ because you want to be very sure that the drug is not toxic before you prescribe it. On the other hand, if you were interested in finding associations between waking fantasy and nighttime dreams, you might be satisfied with $p = .10$, because an erroneous belief in this relationship, while bad for your theories, would not cause great damage to your patient if you were wrong.

You can err on either side. You can reject the null hypothesis and conclude that there is a reliable difference between the two groups when in truth there is none, or you can decide to accept the null hypothesis, claiming that there is no reliable difference between the groups you studied when, in truth, there is one. It all depends where you set the confidence level. Obviously, both extremes need to be avoided. Setting the level too high (e.g., $p = .00001$) and then claiming that there are almost no reliable differences between groups or that almost no interventions cause any changes may, in the long run, be as detrimental to knowledge as setting the level too low (e.g., $p = .20$) and seeing differences and effects when, in fact, there are none.

The basic purpose of inferential statistics is to decide which hypotheses are likely to be correct on the basis of incomplete data (i.e., on the basis of a small sample when the entire population should have been measured to know for sure). We accept the fact that uncertainty is inherent in the scientific enterprise, and our effort is to minimize it. Given this state of affairs, the value of replicating experiments cannot be overemphasized. If you replicate an experiment that yielded a $p = .05$ and again find a $p = .05$, you get a final confidence level of $p = .0025$ ($.05 \times .05 = .0025$). Replicating your own research typically will reduce the list of your publications, but it does wonders for your credibility and eliminates much confusion from the literature.

SAMPLE SIZE

If you only measure one client it is difficult to generalize to the entire population of patients because you don't know whether the one patient is close to the average for the population or happens to be far away from it. If you measure all persons in a population you know for certain what the average and standard deviation are, but measuring all persons of a given population is not only expensive, it is often impossible. The most appropriate number of measurements lies somewhere in between. The more patients you measure, the more confident you become about the true mean and the true standard deviations of the population, but the more expensive your research will be.

How many clients you measure before you are reasonably confident about the results depends, to a large extent, on the strength of the effect you measure. If a disease was 100 percent fatal in the past and the first two patients you treat with a new method both survive, you are reasonably confident that there is an effect. The weaker the effect is that you are studying and the more uncontrollable factors that can muddy the findings, the larger the group of subjects you need to study. Other variables affecting how many subjects you need to study are the levels of measurement you can apply (e.g., ordinal or ratio) and the reliability of these measurements.

CORRELATIONS AND GROUP COMPARISONS

If you have two or more variables and you want to study how they are related, you are doing a correlational analysis. Examples would be to study whether income relates to intelligence, whether the amount of aggression relates to amount of religiosity in the family, or whether the plasma levels of certain neurotransmitters relate to the severity of depression. You can compute certain types of correlations even on ordinal data.

If you compare different groups with each other (e.g., you compare depressives with schizophrenics on some variables), or if you compare the performance of one group over time (e.g., before and after treatment), you are dealing with the analysis of group differences. There can be two or more groups to compare.

There are also mixed methods, where some data are grouped, other data are correlational. For example, you may want to know how academic performance relates to the amount of family discord (correlation) in a group of depressives versus a group of normals (group comparisons).

Groups can be either independent or matched. If the same people are used in both groups (e.g., the same patients before and after treatment), or if pairs of people in the two groups have been selected because they show some of the same important characteristics, you have a matched design. If the matching is done well on all important parameters, matched designs are more powerful than nonmatched designs.

Concerning the power of matched designs, over 50 years ago officials in an English county (Lancashire) wondered whether providing milk in schools would help their students to grow taller. For an entire year the county provided milk for 5,000 students, no milk for another 5,000 students. R. A. Fisher, an eminent statistician of that time, criticized this heroic experiment by showing that simply selecting 50 identical twins from this county and giving the milk to one twin in each pair and not to the other in a matched design would have provided more powerful evidence than giving the milk to 5,000 students in the independent design that was used (Fisher, 1958). Such is the power of good matching.

SELECTING THE RIGHT TEST FOR YOUR DATA

Rejecting the null hypothesis is almost always the goal of your research. (Remember, the null hypothesis states that there is no difference. You almost always want to find a difference.) The test that can do this with the most confidence and with the least amount of data is called the most powerful test. Unfortunately, the more powerful a test, the more basic assumptions it makes about the population. If these assumptions are not met, the conclusions drawn from the statistical tests may be invalid.

By now, statisticians have developed appropriate tests for practically all configurations of data sets. The goal, then, is simply to find the appropriate test for your design and for your level of measurement. This is when it really pays to talk to the statistician before embarking on the study, because small adjustments in your design and your measurements may well let you use more powerful tests thus allowing you to test your hypothesis with far less data.

Explaining your data to the statistician, you may expect to be asked some of the following questions:

1. Is the sample truly random? This means that each individual in the population has an equal chance to get selected, and that having selected one case of the population should not influence the chances of any other case in the population to be selected.

2. How is the trait likely to be distributed in the population? As you have seen, normal distribution is a mathematically defined, complex property. In practice, it means that most cases are near the middle, few cases are at the extremes.

3. How are the variables scaled? (See the discussion of levels of measurement.)

4. Are the populations from which you drew your samples likely to have equal variance, or at least a known ratio between the variances? Also, for some tests, are the effects due to rows and due to columns additive? These two questions are tough ones; your statistician may first have to explain to you what the questions mean before you can answer them. Also, the statistician may have to do some empirical testing on your data to answer these questions unless there is some information available from previous work.

Depending on your answers to these questions, the statistician may decide to use either a parametric or a nonparametric test. *Parameter* means boundary or characteristic. In this context, it means at least normally distributed. The more you know about the characteristics of your variable, the more likely it is that the more powerful parametric tests can be used.

Based on the knowledge discussed so far, you are now ready to discuss your data with a statistician and select the proper tests. What follows here is a list of some tests that are very commonly used. This should give you at least some feeling about what is available or some idea of what people were doing whose research reports you are reading:

Tests of Association

Pearson correlation coefficients. The Pearson correlation co-efficient tests relationships between two variables when the data meet the assumptions for parametric tests.

Spearman correlation coefficients. The Spearman correlation coefficient is a similar test of relationships for (rank ordered) ordinal data that do not meet the assumptions for parametric tests.

Group Tests

t-tests are used if you compare two groups and have parametric data. Depending on your design, you may use the matched-t or the independent-t test.

Analysis of variance (ANOVA). Analysis of variance can be used if you have two or more groups and one or more variables to assess. Analysis of variance (ANOVA) is a complex set of comparisons that can test two or more hypotheses at the same time. For example, assume you select patients randomly for four different treatments and assess their performance before the treatment, after the treatment, and at a one-year follow-up. The ANOVA tests indicate whether there are any significant changes over time, or inherent in the four groups (e.g., one group consistently better than another). Analysis of variance also indicates whether the effects are attributable to an interaction between treatment and passage of time (one group improving more than another over time, or one group getting better over time, another one worse, etc). Doing an ANOVA is complex and usually involves a consultant who is relatively sophisticated in its mechanics.

Nonparametric tests. Nonparametric tests such as the Mann-Whitney U Test, the Wilcoxon matched-pairs-signed-ranks tests, and the Friedman two-way analysis of variance by ranks are clearly described in Siegel (1956). They take the place of the t-test or the analysis of variance when parametric assumptions are not met.

Chi-square. The chi-square test and its many variants are used to treat discontinuous data (nominal or ordinal levels of measurement). Basically, you compare the frequencies you have observed in your experiment with frequencies you had expected and see if there are any significant differences.

Besides the limited number of tests discussed here, there are many others. In mental health work one often uses complex designs that evaluate the effects of many different variables simultaneously, because it is rare that one variable can be isolated by itself for manipulation or study. Most of our phenomena are dependent on a host of variables acting in concert. It is impossible to explain these tests in a short chapter. For reference, names of some of these complex tests are: analysis of covariance, principal components analysis, factor analysis, multiple analysis of variance (MANOVA), and discriminant analysis. Most of us need statisticians to use them, but you should know that many multivariate tests exist.

A serious problem with the complex multivariate tests is the fact that compared with the simple tests they need many more data points (e.g., many more subjects to be measured) before they can be used. Although it is true that the exact number of data points needed to measure an effect depends on many things such as mean differences, standard deviations, and desired confidence limits (discussed early in this chapter), a general, rough rule of thumb is that you need ten times more independent data points than you have variables. Thus, if you want to assess how 20 different variables affect each other, you will need, at the very minimum, to measure these 20 variables in 200 patients. This is probably beyond the beginner's capability. It is better to stick to simple designs and tests until expertise is built up.

MULTIPLE COMPARISONS

You will remember that a significance level of $p = .05$ means that in about one of 20 trials the data could have been selected from a random numbers table with an effect as large or larger than the one reported. Obviously, if you run 40 comparisons on the same data set, it is likely that about two of them will be significant at the .05 level, even if you picked the data from a random numbers table.

With the advent of the computer, analyzing data in many different ways has become easy. Most computer libraries contain almost every test you would ever need, and computers perform most analyses in a matter of seconds. Thus, much data is currently over-analyzed, leading to the problem of finding some spurious statistical significance where there is no real difference.

To guard against the possibility of over-analyzing the data and getting significant results where there are none, special criteria have to be fulfilled if the same data are used for more than one statistical analysis. Any statistician and most statistics books can provide these criteria. You should simply remember that if you know exactly what you are looking for, it is best to analyze each data set only once for that effect, so as not to weaken the confidence levels by multiple comparisons.

Our most important word of advice in this chapter: Discuss your research plans with someone knowledgeable in statistics before you start to collect data. Many a pile of data lies around unanalyzable because the statistician's advice was sought too late, when a slight change in the design of the study could have made the data amenable to study.

Chapter 13

How to Write a Paper for Publication

Writing a scientific article is difficult. It demands work. You are limited by the space that is available in scientific journals and by the time that other scientists are willing to give to reading what you have to say. Therefore, your paper has to have something worthwhile to say, and it has to be clear and brief.

A scientific paper is a communication of facts and ideas, not of feelings. To do its work effectively, it must be clear in thought, simple in expression, and logical in the sequence of its presentation.

To increase the probability that your work will be published and understood, it is important that it be well written. Many of us are like Flaubert, who described his difficulty translating thoughts into writing as follows: "I am like a violinist whose ear is true, but whose fingers refuse to reproduce the sounds he hears within." To write well and easily, you must read examples of good writing, and you must write often.

Braceland (1978) suggests the simple approach: "One simply says what he means in simple, declarative sentences." But Braceland goes on to note that writers too often "take a simple statement, choke it to death with adjectives, put as much as they can into the passive voice, and then embalm it further in polysyllables, making it more un-understandable."

For the beginning mental health researcher who is writing a scientific paper for the first time, it is preferable to undertake a case report or a short, focused review article, rather than attempting a full-scale, original research paper. These less complex tasks will lend themselves better to clear, simple, and straightforward thinking and writing. They will also be more manageable in terms of time and size.

Whether writing a case report or an original article, expect to write and rewrite several drafts. As Braceland (1978) described it accurately:

> Clear, brisk writing is a joy to read. Apparently no courses and no 'how to do it' books make a good writer. Most writing has to be done by ordinary folks like us, writing and rewriting and plugging away, practicing, taking criticism, striking out unnecessary words, and then writing it over again.

In writing an original research article, keep in mind that "the primary aim of a scientific paper is to present, in the simplest possible manner, the results of a particular inquiry and the conclusions which stem from them. *Originality, clarity*, and *brevity* are its three essentials" (Leigh 1975).

You are ready to begin to write only after you have completed your literature review, developed an alphabetized and annotated bibliography, gathered and analyzed your experimental data, and formulated your conclusions. One way to proceed is first to organize all your materials, including relevant literature, methodologies, results, interpretations and conclusions into groupings that will correspond roughly to an introduction, a methods section, a results section, and a discussion section. Having each individual reference, thought, or datum on a separate index card will greatly facilitate this process.

The organization and content of each section will depend to a large extent on the journal to which you are planning to submit your work. Before you start, it will help if you are familiar with the format, content, and organization expected by that journal as reflected both in papers published in it and in its instructions to authors. Usually instructions are found on a front or back page of selected issues.

For each section of your paper, you next develop a topic outline, listing in abbreviated style the thoughts or topics that go into each section and how they follow each other. Keep in mind the following questions in developing your outlines:

> What is the purpose and scope of each section and of each paragraph within that section? How should the paragraphs be best arranged to form a logical sequence? What information and ideas should be included in each paragraph, and how is the information or idea to be introduced and organized? What points need the greatest emphasis? What diagrams and tables will be needed and where? Is it often desirable to prepare tables and diagrams before writing so that you can organize your thoughts and refer to them in the text. What subheadings will help the reader? Often a subheading for each paragraph is helpful to the writer, even if it is deleted in the final paper.

Give some thought to an effective beginning that will capture the reader's interest. For most professionals there is too much to read and too little time in which to read it. The title, the abstract or summary, and the first paragraph or two should be written in such a way as to stimulate the reader's interest. The title, especially, should be brief, descriptive, and informative enough to capture the reader's attention. Likewise, an effective ending with appropriate emphasis and impact will help ensure that the reader will carry your main message away with him.

Working from your topic outline, try to write each section, or the entire paper if it is not too long, at one sitting. Write simply, clearly, and with the first words that come to mind. Assume that you are telling a friend what you have found out in this area. How would you say it? When you have completed the draft, set it aside for a while. Begin to revise the draft only after some days have elapsed. In general, it is well to "write in haste, revise at leisure" (Lucas, 1962).

It will help to review the following before you begin the revision process. What is the study about (its objective)? Why was it done? Why is it relevant? How does it relate to what others have found? What were its essential findings and conclusions?

When you have the draft revised to your satisfaction, ask at least two knowledgeable colleagues to review it critically. You should ask them to be merciless in their criticism; this will pay off in the long run when your paper is being read just as critically by editorial reviewers. Then revise and rewrite again with the criticisms and comments of your two readers in mind.

When you are near a final draft, you should measure your paper against the following checklist. The longer the paper, the more difficult it is to publish. Is each paragraph necessary, relevant, understandable, and in its proper place? Is the connection between paragraphs clear and logical? Are your arguments forcefully developed and taken to their logical conclusion? Are original findings, data, and conclusions sufficiently emphasized? Does the paper include any material irrelevant to its main conclusions? Cut the irrelevant material, even if it is interesting or good prose.

SUBMISSION FOR PUBLICATION

When you have your final draft, once again consult the "Instructions to Authors" page of the journal to which you plan to submit the paper. Have the manuscript organized and typed in the prescribed format. This is especially important with the reference section, which is styled quite differently by different journals.

After you have submitted the final manuscript, you will usually receive an acknowledgment from the editor in about two weeks. Then, be patient. Final word of editorial action taken may not arrive for up to nine months. Rarely is it less than two months.

When you finally hear from the editor, you will usually receive unsigned copies of the reviewers' comments and will be told one of the following:

1. The paper has been accepted unconditionally. This is extremely rare. For example, we understand that in 1985 out of over 1000 papers submitted to the *American Journal of Psychiatry* only three were accepted without revision.
2. The paper has been accepted under condition that it be satisfactorily revised along the lines of the reviewers' criticisms and suggestions.

3. The paper has been neither accepted nor rejected. You are being invited to revise the manuscript along the lines of the reviewers' criticism and resubmit it for further consideration. While this is no guarantee of eventual acceptance, it generally means that the editor and reviewers see merit in the paper and will give it a careful second reading.
4. The paper has been rejected. In such cases further revision and resubmission are neither invited nor warranted. If you feel your paper has merit, it is best to start thinking of another place to submit it.

There are many reasons why a paper may be rejected. Most have to do with its quality, originality, and content. The paper may not be timely, or it may contain no new information. The subject of the paper may not be suitable for the journal in question. The paper may not achieve its stated purpose and goal, or its conclusion may not be supported by the data and results that were presented. The technical format, statistical analyses, or reference style may not be acceptable, or appropriate credit may not have been given for borrowed ideas.

Other significant reasons may have little to do with the quality of the work. These include the volume and quality of other manuscripts; available space in the journal; the journal's format, which may call for a specified proportion of case reports, reviews, original articles, and editorials (Kirkpatrick & Roland, 1977); or the reviewer may have failed to understand or misconstrued the major points of your article. When the latter happens, it is well to bear in mind that the quality and uniformity of reviewers' opinions may be quite variable. But also bear in mind that good writing is rarely misunderstood. If you feel that your paper was misconstrued or inappropriately reviewed, it is occasionally acceptable to write to the editor and politely ask for another review.

If your paper is accepted, feel smug, celebrate, and be prepared to wait again. Anywhere from 2 to 20 months may pass before it appears in print. If your paper is rejected, do not take it personally, since as many as nine out of ten submitted manuscripts are rejected by some journals. If you believe your work has merit, try to improve it further, using the reviewers' comments, and then resubmit it to another journal. You may have to go through this process several times, but don't despair. If it is good, it will eventually be published. As discussed previously, the quality and the value of your work is only one of many factors that affect whether the paper is accepted for publication.

STYLISTIC HINTS

Each writer develops his or her own style of writing over time. Nonetheless, there are fundamental precepts of good writing. Suggestions are included in the appended list of "Do's and Don'ts of Good Writing" (scientific or otherwise) and in articles by Christy (1979), Radovsky (1979), and Crichton (1975) on medical writing. Crichton's article is a superb discussion of what is wrong with most medical writing, and you would do well to start by reading it carefully.

Do's and Don'ts of Good Writing

1. Always decide what you want to say, why, and to whom before you start to write.
2. At the beginning come straight to the point, try to capture your reader's interest by referring to things he or she already knows, and then build on this foundation.
3. Explain new concepts fully.
4. In general, use short, well structured paragraphs.
5. Introduce new topics forcefully in the first sentence of a new paragraph.
6. Use short sentences to introduce a subject or bring a discussion of a topic to a close.
7. Use longer sentences to develop a point; but be sure they are well organized and tightly structured.
8. Omit unnecessary words.
9. Say things as succinctly as is compatible with clarity.
10. When you are trying to rewrite a poor sentence, ask yourself, "What is it I want to say here?"
11. Avoid "etc." at the end of a list. It is better to use "for example" or "including" immediately before giving such a list.

12. Put statements into a positive form if at all possible.
13. Use definite, specific, concrete language.
14. Use simple words; avoid fancy words. For example, use the word *use* instead of *utilize*.
15. Use the active voice whenever possible.
16. Avoid the use of qualifiers unless they are necessary.
17. Do not inject your own opinions and conclusions when you talk about your methods and your results.
18. Avoid foreign words unless they are in common usage.
19. Prefer the standard to the offbeat in choosing words or syntax.
20. Use figures of speech sparingly.
21. Do not overwrite or overstate.
22. Do not explain the obvious.
23. Do not take shortcuts at the cost of clarity.
24. Avoid jargon.

Chapter 14

Writing and Publishing
from a Resident's Point of View

This chapter was written by a psychiatric resident (EJV) who has managed to publish a number of papers during his residency training. It was written independent of the previous chapters and covers some of the same areas, but from a different point of view. It also recounts the publication of an actual case series from beginning to end.

A principal end product of research is a report that allows the researcher to communicate with colleagues. This report should explain what was done, why it was done, how it was done, and what the researcher concluded from the data. Alternatively, if the research consists of a topic review, the report summarizes existing data, reveals trends, and condenses useful information into a short and understandable format.

This chapter reviews the process of writing a scientific article, be it a case report or a review article. Such case reports or reviews seem simple. Don't let this fool you. Neither is a trivial piece of writing, and both can make significant contributions to theoretical formulations and clinical understanding. Each is approached by a series of steps: developing an idea; expanding, refining, and defining the article topic; data gathering; outlining; writing; and submitting for publication. It will at times be necessary to consider several steps simultaneously.

DEVELOPING AN IDEA

Generating a topic for a paper is not difficult. Sources are innumerable in both academic and clinical settings. The beginning of an idea can often develop in conferences, meetings, seminars, rounds, and discussions. Even talking about cases or topics over coffee can be a beginning. Catch phrases can act as tip-offs to an eventual published piece: "This is so unusual it should be published," "I've never heard of a case like that," or "I've never seen anything written about that." Asking colleagues, especially senior clinicians in training centers, can be rewarding. Cases you find intriguing or unusual should make you consider the possibility of a report.

Reading can be an excellent and often overlooked source for developing ideas for research and review articles. In reading, watch for such catch phrases as " . . . however, this aspect has never been formally studied," "more research is needed in this area." Any time you find yourself thinking, "But what about . . . ?" you should consider the possibility that this could lead to a paper. The fiction writers' dictum "read what you write" applies equally well to the mental health researcher. Familiarity with the literature increases the possibilities of developing ideas that can eventually become published.

Another excellent source for a short, well-focused review article is to review the literature on a new drug that particularly interests you about one to two years after its approval by the FDA (or equivalent agency in other countries). Waiting longer than this often results in an unmanageable quantity of data. One can focus on the therapeutic efficacy of the drug itself, on side effects, on untoward or unexpected reactions, or on new or different uses. Clearly, there is an endless supply of topics.

EXPANDING, REFINING, AND DEFINING AN IDEA

The next step is to begin developing data to find out what is known either about cases similar to yours or about the topic you are interested in reviewing. Also find out if there is a place in the literature for your eventual production.

Begin by asking the people around you: attendings, senior clinicians, supervisors, and colleagues. Ask for any knowledge about articles on your topic. Ask the experts what they know. A warning is needed here, however. It has been my experience that these experts can be either extremely helpful or obfuscating. Upon learning why you want to know about the topic in question, they can sometimes overwhelm and submerge you with recommendations, additions, and suggestions. This can lead to the point where you feel you will need a multi-million-dollar, multicenter, placebo-controlled, double-blind, and cross-over study, completely grant funded, to find the answer to your question. When you feel this happening, stop listening. Get the data you want and be on your way. I suggest you read "The Case Report" by King and Roland (1968) to assist in the process of defining an idea and deciding if it is worthy of publication.

DATA GATHERING

Following discussions with colleagues and review of the data you have culled so far, you will develop an idea of what you want to write. Read the material you have so far collected, including the references. References are important. They can direct you to further useful sources — a sort of free search service. Then do a formal literature search (Huth, 1982). Unless there are compelling reasons for a chronologically shorter search, look through the last five years of *Index Medicus, Biological Abstracts, Psychological Abstracts*, etc., whichever are most relevant. Use computerized search services in larger libraries. Ask the reference librarian what is available. Also, if you have a personal computer with a modem, a large number of search services can be subscribed to at very reasonable cost (Hewitt & Chalmers, 1985, a and b).

Continue refining your topic during the literature search. For example, searching "bipolar affective disorders" is simply too large a category to manage. Refine it by searching "bipolar affective disorders" and something else, such as medication, a particular response, a psychological intervention, or the co-occurrence of an additional disorder. Be sure that complete reference data is on your copy as you collect articles (name of journal, volume and issue number, year, month, and pages). This will prevent having to return to the stacks to complete bibliographic data to prepare a list of references.

While you read the material you are collecting, separate the data you think is related to your topic. Underline, write margin notes, or write the information and source on index cards.

OUTLINING

By now your topic is focusing. You also have supporting literature. Since each journal has a slightly different slant in terms of what it publishes and a specific format for how a paper is to be prepared, now make a list of journals to which you would like to submit your paper (Kirkpatrick & Roland, 1977). I recommend a list of four to six journals. Most beginning writers intend to be accepted by one of the major journals. Wrong. I speak from painful experience. It is easier to be published initially in the slightly less prestigious journals. The experience gained is valuable for later submissions to progressively better known publications.

Now for an easy part. Get one or two recent issues of each journal on your list. Read their case reports or short reviews. They can be used as guides for setting up your own paper. They can also give you an idea about the preferred format of each journal: length and precision of abstract, general introduction length, average content of a case report, and general style for review articles. Additionally, read the "Instructions for Authors" page of each journal before writing. These pages can occasionally define a format for you. Also, be aware that there exist reference works for uniform requirements and standards for biomedical writing (International Committee of Medical Journal Editors, 1982; Barclay et al., 1981; Publication Manual of the American Psychological Association, 1983).

With your topic in mind, references in hand, and a general idea of how the paper should flow, it is time to outline. You probably hate outlining. However, a good outline helps you to keep focused. A good outline can practically write itself.

Separate the various portions of your paper, for example, introduction, methods, results, and discussion; or perhaps introduction, biological, psychological, social, and other categories, and a summary for a review article. Write a separate outline for each portion. Be aware that introductions should be short and concise. It was a tradition of nineteenth-century American biomedical writing to review all extant world literature in an introduction. No longer. Limit introductions to a few paragraphs.

In case reports, present only the relevant data. There is necessarily some value judgment involved, but normally data that are not clearly related to the case or to the issue involved need not be included. If readers are sufficiently interested, they may write to the author. Also remember that automated chemistry profiles may vary between hospitals, depending on their laboratory equipment. Therefore, do not report that "Profile x was within normal limits." If germane to the case, state that values a, b, c, etc., were normal. With reviews, use associated review articles for references rather than repeating all of their work. This saves time and space, and it increases the clarity of your paper.

Conclusions (in case reports) and summarizing statements (in review articles) need also be outlined. Perhaps several conclusions or statements can be drawn. Each deserves a separate outline entry, so they do not get lost in the writing.

WRITING

The very word strikes fear in the hearts of beginners. It needn't. Just as you now realize that there is a process to developing and honing a topic for a paper, so is there a process for writing. There are easily available examples and guides (Day, 1983; King, 1978; Leigh, 1975). The following suggestions seem most useful for the beginner.

Good scientific writing is clear, crisp, and concise. Unfortunately, most writers make consistent errors. I recommend you read Michael Crichton's *"Medical Obfuscation: Structure and Function"* (1975) for a discussion of the most glaring faults.

A problem for most beginning writers is being overinclusive. Remember that you are writing a case report or focused review. You need not rewrite all known information about your topic. However, if you must write everything, do so. Then edit most of it away later.

Follow professional writing rules. Use simple sentences. Try not to begin or end a sentence with a preposition. Simple words are better than difficult words. Get rid of any word that does not contribute to your paper. Reread a case study or review that you found enjoyable; doubtless it will be clear, crisp, and concise.

Note also that it will have little extraneous detail, redundancy, or unnecessary complexity.

I recommend you write each section of your paper at one sitting, perhaps a section per day. When you are finished, set the whole thing aside for about a week. After some distance and separation, read, rewrite, and edit your first draft. Free-lance writers say that a good form for an article is to "tell them what you're going to tell them, then tell them, then tell them what you just told them." This approach applies to the case report, corresponding to the introduction, body, and discussion respectively, and for the review article, to the introduction, review proper, and summary.

During editing, remember that your writing is not cast in stone. Portions may be interchanged if this improves the flow of ideas. Simplify whenever possible. Eliminate repetition. This rewriting and editing yields a second draft.

Set your paper aside again. Then edit for the final draft: pay attention to fine detail, grammar, punctuation, smoothness of flow, simplicity of structure, and precision and relatedness of paragraph structure.

As an article nears completion, anxiety increases. One of the mechanisms I've seen used to bind this anxiety is the never-ending rewrite. Another person, at some point, will read your paper. It should be now. Ask a colleague to review it. Choose someone who has been published, if possible. When this reviewer's comments are in, evaluate the comments and incorporate them into your paper if they are appropriate.

Review your article one last time, do not rewrite it. Check for accuracy of reference citations. Make sure it meets the submission requirements of the journal you will submit it to. Make sure the final draft is clean and legible.

SUBMITTING FOR PUBLICATION

Your paper is finished, ready to be submitted. Prepare a cover letter and address it to the appropriate editor. This information is on the "Instructions for Authors" page. Also, some journals require a statement of transfer of copyright in the cover letter. Check the instructions for the required wording.

A cover letter, like your article, should be clear and concise. It is enough to say that you are submitting the enclosed paper (give title) for publication in (name of journal). A brief comment on timeliness or appropriateness of your paper for the particular journal is often good form.

Seal it up, send it out, and wait, often up to six months. Three things can happen: (1) It can be unconditionally accepted. This is rare. If it happens — congratulations! (2) It can be rejected. If this happens, make any necessary changes required to make it meet requirements for the next journal on your list and send it out. (3) It can be returned with recommendations for changes. Here you have several options. You can make the changes (if you agree with them) and resubmit it to the same journal. You can let the paper stand as is and submit it to another journal. Or you can make the changes and submit it to a different journal. In any case, use the reviewer's comments as constructive commentary. In a number of cases, they can point out flaws in an otherwise good paper. Finally, remember that many papers go through several rejections before finally being accepted.

REPORT OF A CASE SERIES

In order to increase the utility of this chapter, I present here a blow-by-blow account of how one case report came to publication.

At the end of my first year of residency training, I was bombarded by senior residents trying to find therapists to whom they could transfer cases. I listened to many presentations. One catch phrase captured my attention: " . . . actually, she's a reportable case. I just never got around to it." I immediately picked up a case of opioid-responsive restless legs syndrome, a sleep disorder I had never heard of at the time.

After reviewing the case, I looked through a few of the standard sleep disorders textbooks without much gain. I then spoke with the director of the sleep disorders center. He was quite interested. In fact, he also had such a case of restless legs syndrome which was being effectively treated with an opioid. I then spoke with several other residents, and one knew of yet another case she'd seen while on the consultation service. None of us, however, were aware of any literature concerning this aspect of restless legs.

A MEDLINE search of the literature and a review of recent issues of the *Index Medicus* yielded 48 references. Nineteen of these were pertinent to our interest. The references contained in these sources yielded 10 additional articles. The review of this literature proved that we did indeed have sufficiently unusual case material to warrant a report.

We opted to collaborate on a multiple case report. We reviewed our three cases, and each of us then wrote a rough draft report. Since the treatment modality was unusual, it was decided early that the *American Journal of Psychiatry* would be our first target journal. A word limit (noted in the Information for Contributors) necessitated limiting the length of the case reports. The following is the first draft of case number one.

Ms. A. is a 58-year-old Caucasian woman who first presented to our psychiatry service in 1964 with a situational depression. She also complained of lower leg aches since her second pregnancy in 1956, which continued except for a three year period post-partum. These aches were steady, non-throbbing, and poorly localized and occurred upon retiring, during daytime rest and interrupted sleep. Relief was obtained by pacing. Neurologic exams, skin and muscle biopsies were normal.

Ms. A. was also addicted to meperidine, codeine, and pentazocine at various times between 1968 and 1972. During that period her leg aches persisted and she had chronic insomnia. In 1972, after detoxification from pentazocine, she was treated with amitriptyline 150 mg qd for atypical depression. An empirical trial of methadone 10 mg bid brought relief of her leg discomforts within 4 days and her sleep improved. Polysomnography (without medications) revealed a series of repeated myoclonic jerking following Stage 2 sleep which caused awakenings with achy lower legs requiring pacing for up to one half hour.

Since 1972 no further drug abuse has been noted and Ms. A. has experienced continued relief from restless legs with methadone 10 mg qhs, with recurrences of symptoms if the dose is decreased. Intermittent courses of amitriptyline for recurrent depressions have not affected the restless leg symptoms.

This first draft is difficult to read, does not flow well, and is grammatically flawed. We reviewed and edited each other's reports. The second draft of case number one follows. Note that it certainly is easier to read and understand.

> Ms. A. is a 58-year-old Caucasian woman who first presented to the psychiatry service in 1964 with a situational depression. At that time she complained of lower leg aches since her second pregnancy in 1956. Except for a three-year period post-partum, these aches were continuous and described as steady, non-throbbing, and poorly localized, occurring upon retiring and during daytime rest and during sleep interruptions. Relief was obtained by pacing. Neurologic examinations, skin and muscle biopsies were normal.
>
> Ms. A. has a history of meperidine and codeine abuse and was addicted to pentazocine (200-600 mg IM qd) at various times between 1968 and 1972. Although somewhat improved by these medications, her leg aches persisted and she had chronic difficulties maintaining sleep. In 1972, after detoxification from pentazocine, she was treated with amitriptyline 150 mg qd for atypical depression. An empirical trial of methadone 10 mg b.i.d. brought relief of her leg discomforts within 4 days and her sleep improved. Polysomnography (without medications) revealed a series of repeated periodic leg movements following Stage 2 sleep, which caused awakenings with achy lower legs requiring pacing for up to one half hour.
>
> Since 1972 no further drug abuse has been noted, and Ms. A. has experienced continued relief from restless legs with methadone 10 mg qhs, but the symptoms recur whenever the dose is decreased. Intermittent courses of amitriptyline for recurrent depression have not affected the restless leg symptoms.

A third rewrite is the one that eventually appeared in print, the only changes being those suggested by the formal reviewers.

(The case report is reprinted in its entirety at the end of this chapter.*)

Similar processes occurred for the introduction and discussion portions of the paper. Only ten references were cited in the final version, because of a limit set by the publisher. More important, however, this demonstrates that it is possible to use far fewer references than you have at hand.

The paper was then submitted to the editor of the *American Journal of Psychiatry*. Printing the entire submitted paper here would be too lengthy. I have reproduced the three reviewers' comments. This will give you an idea of their concerns and recommendations.

> REVIEWER #1: This clinical report offers three uncontrolled case histories supporting the use of low-dose narcotics in the successful treatment of restless legs syndrome, a disorder resulting in chronic sleep disturbance. The disorder seems to appear in middle-aged individuals who may have a past history of drug abuse or serious medical illness, but the etiology or pathophysiological mechanism of the disorder are not understood. Knowledge of the disorder could be helpful to the practicing psychiatrist and further research is needed. This paper would make an excellent clinical report in the short Clinical and Research Reports section, but it must be shortened to fit the 1300 word requirement. It would also be helpful to discuss any tentative pathophysiological mechanisms and etiological explanations for the disorder and what action opiates might play in symptom relief.

> REVIEWER #2: It is to be hoped that the success of treating these three patients with opioid drugs does not represent some subtle transference manifestation. That seems unlikely. In retrospect it might have been useful to have had periods of placebo use to control for that. In case one, polysomnography revealed "leg movements following Stage 2 sleep." It's unclear to this reviewer exactly what the authors mean. Did the leg movements start during Stage 2

Amer. J. Psychiatry, 141 (8):993-995, 1984, the American Psychiatric Association. Reprinted by permission.

sleep and cause the awakenings, or did they start immediately after the awakening? If so, what is actually meant as the cause of awakenings? It might be of interest to be more precise in case three as well with regard to the actual stage and phase of sleep during which the leg movements occurred.

REVIEWER #3: These are important clinical observations which could be of great benefit to patients with these very disturbing disorders. I recommend publication if the authors could shorten it to the 1300 word format and include the following cautions.

Diagnosis was made on the basis of a typical clinical history. Only one subject was apparently evaluated by polysomnography. In this particular case, the authors should clarify their observations. It is not clear from the present description when the periodic leg movement occurred. Since no well established therapies currently exist to treat these vexing problems, the present observations that opiates may be helpful are particularly important. I would suggest that the write-up include specific remarks recommending future double-blind, carefully controlled studies of opiates in this disorder. Furthermore, the article should not be subject to misinterpretation or encourage careless or unscrupulous use of opiates in this or other disorders in the future. The long-term benefits of this therapy are obviously unknown at this time, but we have every reason to believe that there could be serious problems with misuse of opiates. I am concerned that some practitioners may opt to use these drugs in patients with complaints of insomnia, but without having established the proper diagnosis of nocturnal myoclonus and without adequate monitoring and evaluation. Perhaps these drugs should only be used under research control in patients who have been diagnosed and followed in a research sleep disorders center.

The article was shortened to meet the required word limitation. The final version was submitted with a 1210 word count. The polysomnographic findings were clarified. The discussion of etiology and pathophysiology was expanded. Finally, in response to the concerns of reviewer #3, the last sentence was added.

So there you have it — a quick review of the process by which you begin with an idea and end with a published paper. The process can be approached in a stepwise fashion and thereby made manageable. Any unresolved questions can be answered by reading the appropriate references. All that's left now is to do it.

CASE REPORT

Response to Opioids in Three Patients With Restless Legs Syndrome

Paula T. Trzepacz, MD
E. Jeffrey Violette, MD
Michael J. Sateia, MD

SUMMARY. Three patients with restless legs syndrome, two of whom also had nocturnal myoclonus, responded well to treatment with low doses of opioids. The pathophysiology of the syndrome and the mechanism of opioids' therapeutic action are discussed.
(Am J Psychiatry 141:993-995, 1984)

Restless legs syndrome has been described intermittently in the medical literature since the 1800s. Named by Ebkom in 1944, restless legs syndrome is a dysesthesia described as creeping, crawling, prickly, or restless feelings deep in the leg muscles.[1-3] Patients with this disorder may also complain of leg aches.

Received July 25, 1983; revised Feb. 13, 1984; accepted March 5, 1984. From the Sleep Disorders Center and the Department of Psychiatry, Dartmouth Medical School, Hanover, N.H. Address reprint requests to Dr. Trzepacz, Western Psychiatric Institute and Clinic, University of Pittsburgh, 3811 O'Hara St., Pittsburgh, PA 15213.

These sensations are worse when the patient is resting, especially on retiring for the night, leading to chronic insomnia. Relief usually occurs only when the patient responds to an irresistible urge to walk or move the limbs. The syndrome is often associated with periodic movements of sleep, also called nocturnal myoclonus.[4]

Treatments for this syndrome include administration of vasodilating drugs, iron, folate, vitamin E, and clonazepam.[4,5] All have met with varying degrees of success. Occasionally, relief occurs on treatment of an associated disorder such as anemia, uremia, diabetes, nocturnal myoclonus, cancer, or avitaminosis. In addition, there is a familial form with demonstrable evidence of motor neuron disease.[2]

We describe three patients with restless legs syndrome who responded to treatment with an opioid. Two of these three patients were studied with polysomnography.

CASE REPORTS

Case 1. Ms. A, a 58-year-old woman, first appeared at the psychiatry service 20 years earlier with a situational depression. At that time she also complained of poorly localized, nonthrobbing aches in her lower legs that had begun during a pregnancy 8 years before. Except for a 3-year period after the pregnancy, the aches had occurred each day during her daytime rest, when she retired for the night, and when her sleep was interrupted. She was able to obtain relief by pacing. Results of neurologic examinations and skin and muscle biopsies were normal.

Four years after her first visit she began to abuse meperidine and codeine intermittently and became addicted to pentazocine while taking 200-600 mg i.m. once a day. Her leg aches persisted, although they were somewhat improved, and she had chronic difficulty remaining asleep. Four years later, after detoxification from pentazocine, she was treated with 150 mg/day of amitriptyline for an atypical depression. An empirical trial of 10 mg b.i.d. of methadone brought relief of her leg discomfort within 4 days, and her sleep improved. Polysomnography without medication revealed a series of repeated nocturnal myoclonus during stage 2 sleep. She intermittently awakened following the periodic movements and reported having achy lower legs. A half-hour of pacing brought relief.

Since the detoxification admission, Ms. A has experienced continued relief from the restless legs syndrome while taking 10 mg h.s. of methadone and has not abused other drugs. Her symptoms recurred when the dose was decreased. Intermittent courses of amitriptyline for recurrent depression did not affect the restless legs syndrome.

Case 2. The renal dialysis unit requested psychiatric consultation for Mr. B, a 47-year-old man, for evaluation of depression and difficulty in sleeping. He had had diabetes with sensory polyneuropathy, for which he took insulin, for 21 years, and he suffered from renal failure (for which he underwent hemodialysis), anemia, and atherosclerotic cardiovascular disease.

Our consultation showed that Mr. B had an adjustment disorder but not a major depression. He complained of difficulty in initiating and maintaining sleep and of daytime fatigue that forced him to take a nap on days he received dialysis. He denied experiencing nocturnal angina. His insomnia was associated with restless feelings in his legs that made it necessary for him to pace in order to "tire out" his legs. His legs ached in the morning, but this was a different feeling from that of his diabetic polyneuropathy. We diagnosed restless legs syndrome; nocturnal myoclonus was suggested by his history, but it was not documented by polysomnography.

A trial of d-α-vitamin E did not relieve his symptoms. When 2.5 mg h.s. of oxycodone was added, his sleep improved and the symptoms disappeared. Two months after oxycodone treatment began, he underwent renal transplant and the oxycodone was stopped. After the operation, his insomnia and symptoms of restless legs syndrome were gone, although his diabetic paresthesias continued. His serum creatinine level, which before the operation was 8.1 mg/dl, dropped to 1.2 mg/dl and his anemia also improved.

Case 3. Mr. C, a 54-year-old man, was evaluated at the center for 10 to 12 years of difficulty initiating and maintaining sleep and for symptoms of restless legs syndrome. Previous treatments with carbamazepine, clonazepam, and chloral hydrate were unsuccessful. His symptoms improved somewhat during treatment

with 100 mg h.s. of imipramine and with a combination of amitriptyline and L-tryptophan.

Because of his symptoms, he found lying in bed intolerable
and falling asleep difficult. During his multiple night awakenings
the sensation of restlessness recurred so that he got at most 1-2
hours of sleep a night. His spouse observed repetitive leg movements during his sleep.

Polysomnography revealed multiple episodes of nocturnal
myoclonus during stages 1 and 2; his sleep cycles culminated in
his awakening and complaining of having restless legs. A neurologic exam revealed decreased deep-tendon reflexes in both legs
and normal peripheral motor and sensory nerve conductions.

A repeated trial of clonazepam did not alleviate his symptoms.
However, 50 to 100 mg/day of imipramine afforded some improvement, especially in sleep maintenance. When 2.5 mg h.s.
of oxycodone was added to the imipramine the symptoms of restless legs syndrome cleared remarkably and sleep interruptions
became rare. The next 25 months were virtually symptom-free
except for an inexplicable brief period of poorer response. In
addition, discontinuation of either drug results in exacerbation of
the symptoms.

DISCUSSION

In 1960, Ebkom[1] made reference to the cautious use of narcot-
ics in the treatment of restless legs syndrome. Our three patients,
one of whom suffered for 10 years, were relieved of restless legs
syndrome by administration of a stable, low daily dose of a po-
tent opioid alone or in combination with a tricyclic. One patient
had previously been addicted to higher doses of opioids, which
suggests that the efficacy of opioids in restless legs syndrome
may be related to dose and that only lower doses are therapeutic.

Ms. A, whose onset of restless legs syndrome was during
pregnancy, and Mr. C both had longstanding symptoms unattri-
butable to any other condition. Both showed polysomnographic
evidence of nocturnal myoclonus largely confined to stage 2
sleep, although Mr. C also exhibited evidence during stage 1
sleep; neither showed evidence during stage 3, stage 4, or REM
sleep. This specificity of sleep stage is consistent with previous

reports,[6] but the pathophysiological significance is unknown. The recurrent transitions in Ms. A and Mr. C from nocturnal myoclonus to restless legs syndrome immediately on awakening suggests that the two disorders may be the same entity with variable expression depending on the state of consciousness. Mr. C experienced nocturnal myoclonus in a crescendo pattern before his episodes of restless legs syndrome.

In contrast, Mr. B experienced restless legs syndrome together with disorders known to be associated with the syndrome – uremia, anemia, and diabetic peripheral neuropathy[4] – about 6 months after the onset of renal failure and the beginning of dialysis. An association between restless legs syndrome and peripheral nerve damage, as evidenced by decreased motor nerve conduction, has been reported in uremic patients, some of whom reported worsening symptoms as their renal status deteriorated.[3] Following renal transplantation and normalization of his renal function, Mr. B reported complete resolution of his restless legs syndrome despite continued symptoms of diabetic sensory neuropathy.[5] This finding supports the view that the pathophysiology of restless legs syndrome may be in the lower motor neuron.[2,3]

Combined treatment with a tricyclic and an opioid was successful with both Ms. A and Mr. C; Ms. A also had long periods of symptom remission while taking only the opioid. In contrast, others[7,8] have reported cases of myoclonus, with and without restless legs, that were caused by amitriptyline and clomipramine.

The specificity of the therapeutic effect we observed is uncertain. If it is mediated by the neurons, it is unclear if it is a central or a peripheral effect. We would not expect opioid action directly on skeletal muscle or peripheral nerve. Morphine-induced peripheral vasodilation due to decreased α-adrenergic tone may be a result of reduced CNS sympathetic efferent discharges.[9] Successful treatment of restless legs syndrome and nocturnal myoclonus with phenoxybenzamine in a patient with documented peripheral sympathetic overactivity[10] supports a possible vasodilatory mechanism of action for opioid-responsive restless legs syndrome.

Alternatively, exogenous opioids might act on opiate receptors in the spinal cord, brainstem, or both, to modulate afferent stimuli in patients whose nocturnal myoclonus might be viewed as a response to a sensory (afferent) disturbance.

Thus, neither the pathophysiology of restless legs syndrome nor the mechanism of therapeutic action of opioids in relieving such symptoms is known. Our clinical observations require future double-blind controlled studies of the use of opioids for treating this disorder. Given the major risk for abuse and the danger of addiction, we recommended using opioids in the treatment of restless legs syndrome only after careful evaluation and diagnosis in a sleep disorders center.

REFERENCES

1. Ebkom KA: Restless legs syndrome. Neurology 10:868-873, 1960

2. Frankel BL, Patten BM, Gillin JC: Restless legs syndrome: sleep electroencephalographic and neurologic findings. JAMA 230:1302-1303, 1974

3. Callaghan N: Restless legs syndrome in uremic neuropathy. Neurology 16:359-361, 1966

4. Coleman RM: Periodic movements in sleep and restless legs syndrome, in *Sleeping and Waking Disorders*. Edited by Guilleminault C. Menlo Park, Calif, Addison-Wesley, 1982

5. Ayres S, Mihan R: Nocturnal leg cramps: a progress report on response to vitamin E. South Med J 67:1308-1312, 1974

6. Lugaresi E, Coccagna G, Berti-Ceroni G, et al.: Restless legs syndrome and nocturnal myoclonus, in The Abnormalities of Sleep in Man: Proceedings of the 15th European Meeting on Electroencephalography, Bologna, 1967. Edited by Gastaut H, Lugaresi E, Berti-Ceroni G, et al. Bologna, Italy, Aulo Gassi Editore, 1968

7. Lippmann S, Moskovitz R, O'Tuama L: Tricyclic-induced myoclonus. Am J. Psychiatry 134:90-91, 1977

8. Insel TR, Roy BF, Cohen RM, et al.: Possible developments of the serotonin syndrome in man. Am J Psychiatry 139:954-955, 1982

9. Zelis R, Mansour EJ, Capone RJ, et al.: The cardiovascular effects of morphine. J. Clin Invest 54:1247-1258, 1974

10. Ware JC, Pittard JT, Blumoff RL: Treatment of sleep related myoclonus with an alpha receptor blocker, in Sleep Research Abstracts, vol 10. Edited by Chase MH. Los Angeles, Brain Research Institute, 1981

References

MENTAL HEALTH

CHAPTER 1 – WHY SHOULD YOU DO RESEARCH?

Brown, B. S. Crisis in Mental Health Research. *Am J Psychiatry*, 134(2):113-120, 1977.

Sainsbury, P. and N. Kreitman (Eds.). *Methods of Psychiatric Research: An Introduction For Clinical Psychiatrists, Second Edition*. London and New York: Oxford University Press, 1975.

CHAPTER 2 – HOW HAS PSYCHIATRIC RESEARCH BEEN DONE?

Foulds, G. A. and A. Bedord. Hierachy of classes of personal illness. *Psychol Med,* 5(2):181-192, 1975.

Strauss, J. S. and H. Hafez. Clinical questions and "real" research. *Am J Psychiatry,* 138: 1592-1597, 1981.

CHAPTER 3 – HOW TO SEE EACH PATIENT AS AN EXPERIMENT

Houtler, B. D. and H. Rosenberg. The retrospective baseline in single case experiments. *The Behavior Therapist* 8:97-98, 1985.

CHAPTER 4 – ETHICAL ISSUES IN MENTAL HEALTH RESEARCH

Declaration of Helsinki: Recommendations Guiding Medical Doctors in Biomedical Research Involving Human Subjects. *WHO Chronical,* 19:31-32, January 1965.

Nuremberg Code. In: *Trials of War Criminals Before The Nur-*

emberg *Military Tribunals Under Control Council Law No. 10, Volume 2.* Washington, D.C.: U.S. Government Printing Office, 181-182, 1949.

CHAPTER 8 – HOW TO MATCH RESEARCH DESIGN TO RESEARCH QUESTION

Postman, L., Bruner, J. S. and E. McGinnies. Personal values as selective factors in perception. *J Abn Soc Psychol* 43:142-154, 1948. Cited in Osgood *Methods and Theory in Experimental Psychology.* New York: Oxford University Press, 1953.

Rosenthal, R. *Experimenter Effects in Behavioral Research.* New York: Appleton-Century-Crofts, 1966.

CHAPTER 9 – HOW TO SELECT THE VARIABLES TO BE STUDIED

Beck, A. T., Ward, C. H., Mendelson, M., Mock, J., Erbaugh, J. K. An inventory for measuring depression. *Arch Gen Psychiatry* 4:561-571, 1961.

Buros, O.K. *Tests in Print II.* Highland Park, NJ: The Gryphon Press, 1974.

Hamilton, M. Development of a rating scale for primary depressive illness. *Brit J Soc Clin Psychol,* 6:278-296, 1967.

Hargreaves, W. A., Attkisson, C. C. Sorensen, J. E. (Eds.). *Resource Materials For Community Mental Health Education.* Rockville, MD: Department of HEW, PHS, ADAMHA, NIMH, 1977.

Millon, T., Diesenhaus, H. I. *Research Methods in Psychopathology.* New York: John Wiley & Sons, Inc., 1972.

Nunnally, J. C. Overview of psychological measurement in the clinical diagnosis of mental disorders. Wolman, B. B. (Ed.). New York: Plenum Press, 97-146, 1978.

Raskin, A., Brook, T. A. Sensitivity of rating scales completed by psychiatrists, nurses, and patients to antidepressant drug effects. *J Psychiatric Research,* 13(1):31-41, 1976.

Research and Education Association. *Handbook of Psychiatric Rating Scales.* New York: REA, 1981.

Sweetland, R. C. and Keyser, D. J. *Tests.* Kansas City: Test Corporation of America, 1983.

Winget, C. and Kramer, M. *Dimensions of Dreams.* Gainesville, FL: University Presses of Florida, 1979.

CHAPTER 10—FREQUENTLY USED ASSESSMENT DEVICES

Dahlstrom, W. B., Welsh, G. S. and Dahlstrom, L. An MMPI handbook, Volume 2: Research Applications. Minneapolis, MN: University of Minnesota Press, 1975.
Newmark, C. S. (Ed.). *Major Psychological Assessment Instruments.* Boston: Allyn & Bacon, 1985.

CHAPTER 11—HOW TO CARRY THROUGH YOUR RESEARCH PROJECT

CHAPTER 12—HOW TO ANALYZE YOUR RESULTS

Fisher, R. A. Statistical methods for research workers, edition 13. New York: Hafuer Publishing, Inc., 1958.
Holmes, T. H., Rahe, R. H. Social readjustment rating scale. *J Psychosom,* 11:213, 1967.
Siegel, S. *Nonparametric Methods for the Behavioral Sciences.* New York: McGraw-Hill, 1956.

CHAPTER 13—HOW TO WRITE A PAPER FOR PUBLICATION

Braceland, E. J. On editing the journal: ave atque vale. *Am J Psychiatry,* 135:1148-1155, 1978.
Christy, N. P. English is our second language. *N Engl J Medicine,* 300:979-981, 1979.
Criston, M. Medical obfuscation: structure and function. *N Engl J Medicine,* 293:1257-1259, 1975.
Kirkpatrick, R. A. and Roland, C. G. How to decide where to submit a manuscript. *Resident and Staff Physician,* 87-92, 1977.
Leigh, D. How to write a scientific paper. Chapter 18 in Sainsbury, P., Kreitman, N. (Eds.). *Methods of Psychiatric Research, Second Edition.* London: Oxford University Press, 1975.
Lucas, R. *Style.* New York: Collier Books, 1962.

Radovsky, S. S. Medical writing: another look. *N Engl J Medicine,* 301:131-134, 1979.

CHAPTER 14 – WRITING AND PUBLISHING FROM A RESIDENT'S POINT OF VIEW

American Psychological Association, *Publication Manual of.* Third Edition. Washington, D.C.: American Psychological Association, 1983.

Barclay, W. R., Southgate, T. and Mayo R. W. (Eds.). *Manual for Authors and Editors: Editorial Style and Manuscript Preparation.* Los Altos: Lange Medical Publishers, 1981.

Crichton, M. Medical obfuscation: structure and function. *N Engl J Medicine,* 293:1257-1259, 1975.

Day, R. A. How to write and publish a scientific paper, second edition. Philadelphia: ISI Press, 1983.

Hewitt, P. and Chalmers, T. C. Using Medline to peruse the literature. *Controlled Clinical Trials,* 6:75-83, 1985a.

Hewitt, P. and Chalmers, T. C. Perusing the literature: methods of accessing Medline and related databses. *Controlled Clinical Trials,* 6:186-177, 1985b.

Huth, E. J. *How to Write and Publish Papers in the Medical Sciences.* Philadelphia: ISI Press, 1982.

King, L. S. and Roland C. G. The case report. In: *Scientific Writing.* Chicago: American Medical Association, 1968.

King, R. S. *Why Not Say It Clearly: A Guide to Scientific Writing.* Boston: Little Brown & Co., 1978.

Kirkpatrick, R. A. and Roland, C. G. How to decide where to submit a manuscript. *Resident and Staff Physician,* 23:87-92, 1977.

Leigh, D. How to write a scientific paper. Chapter 18 in Sainbury, P. and N. Kreitman (Eds.). *Methods of Psychiatric Research, Second Edition.* London: Oxford University Press, 1975.

Medical Journal Editors, International Committee of. Uniform requirements for manuscripts submitted to biomedical journals. *Annals Int Med,* 96-766-771, 1982.

Appendix 1

The Nuremberg Code

THE PROOF AS TO WAR CRIMES
AND CRIMES AGAINST HUMANITY

Judged by any standard of proof the record clearly shows the commission of war crimes and crimes against humanity substantially as alleged in counts two and three of the indictment. Beginning with the outbreak of World War II criminal medical experiments on non-German nationals, both prisoners of war and civilians, including Jews and "asocial" persons, were carried out on a large scale in Germany and the occupied countries. These experiments were not the isolated and casual acts of individual doctors and scientists working solely on their own responsibility, but were the product of coordinated policy-making and planning at high governmental, military, and Nazi Party levels, conducted as an integral part of the total war effort. They were ordered, sanctioned, permitted, or approved by persons in positions of authority who under all principles of law were under the duty to know about these things and to take steps to terminate or prevent them.

PERMISSIBLE MEDICAL EXPERIMENTS

The great weight of evidence before us is to the effect that certain types of medical experiments on human beings, when kept within reasonably well-defined bounds, conform to the eth-

Reprinted from *Trials of War Criminals before the Nuremberg Military Tribunals under Control Council Law No. 10*, vol. 2 (Washington, D.C.: U.S. Government Printing Office, 1949), pp. 181-182.

ics of the medical profession generally. The protagonists of the practice of human experimentation justify their views on the basis that such experiments yield results for the good of society that are unprocurable by other methods or means of study. All agree, however, that certain basic principles must be observed in order to satisfy moral, ethical and legal concepts:

1. The voluntary consent of the human subject is absolutely essential.

This means that the person involved should have legal capacity to give consent; should be so situated as to be able to exercise free power of choice, without the intervention of any element of force, fraud, deceit, duress, over-reaching, or other ulterior form of constraint or coercion; and should have sufficient knowledge and comprehension of the elements of the subject matter involved as to enable him to make an understanding and enlightened decision. This latter element requires that before the acceptance of an affirmative decision by the experimental subject there should be made known to him the nature, duration, and purpose of the experiment; the method and means by which it is to be conducted; all inconveniences and hazards reasonably to be expected; and the effects upon his health or person which may possibly come from his participation in the experiment.

The duty and responsibility for ascertaining the quality of the consent rests upon each individual who initiates, directs or engages in the experiment. It is a personal duty and responsibility which may not be delegated to another with impunity.

2. The experiment should be such as to yield fruitful results for the good of society, unprocurable by other methods or means of study, and not random and unnecessary in nature.

3. The experiment should be so designed and based on the results of animal experimentation and a knowledge of the natural history of the disease or other problem under study that the anticipated results will justify the performance of the experiment.

4. The experiment should be so conducted as to avoid all unnecessary physical and mental suffering and injury.

5. No experiment should be conducted where there is an a priori reason to believe that death or disabling injury will occur; except, perhaps, in those experiments where the experimental physicians also serve as subjects.

6. The degree of risk to be taken should never exceed that determined by the humanitarian importance of the problem to be solved by the experiment.

7. Proper preparations should be made and adequate facilities provided to protect the experimental subject against even remote possibilities of injury, disability, or death.

8. The experiment should be conducted only by scientifically qualified persons. The highest degree of skill and care should be required through all stages of the experiment of those who conduct or engage in the experiment.

9. During the course of the experiment the human subject should be at liberty to bring the experiment to an end if he has reached the physical or mental state where continuation of the experiment seems to him to be impossible.

10. During the course of the experiment the scientist in charge must be prepared to terminate the experiment at any stage, if he has probable cause to believe, in the exercise of the good faith, superior skill and careful judgment required of him that a continuation of the experiment is likely to result in injury, disability, or death to the experimental subject.

Appendix 2

Declaration of Helsinki: Recommendations Guiding Physicians in Biomedical Research Involving Human Subjects

INTRODUCTION

It is the mission of the physician to safeguard the health of the people. His or her knowledge and conscience are dedicated to the fulfillment of this mission.

The Declaration of Geneva of the World Medical Association binds the physician with the words, "The health of my patient will be my first consideration," and the International Code of Medical Ethics declares that, "A physican shall act only in the patient's interest when providing medical care which might have the effect of weakening the physical and mental condition of the patient."

The purpose of biomedical research involving human subjects must be to improve diagnostic, therapeutic and prophylactic procedures and the understanding of the aetiology and pathogenesis of disease.

In current medical practice most diagnostic, therapeutic or prophylactic procedures involve hazards. This applies especially to biomedical research.

Adopted by the 18th World Medical Assembly, Helsinki, Finland, 1964 amended by the 29th World Medical Assembly, Tokyo, Japan, October, 1975, and the 35th World Medical Assembly, Venice, Italy, October 1983. Reprinted by permission of the World Medical Association.

Medical progress is based on research which ultimately must rest in part on experimentation involving human subjects.

In the field of biomedical research a fundamental distinction must be recognized between medical research in which the aim is essentially diagnostic or therapeutic for a patient, and medical research, the essential object of which is purely scientific and without implying direct diagnostic or therapeutic value to the person subjected to the research.

Special caution must be exercised in the conduct of research which may affect the environment, and the welfare of animals used for research must be respected.

Because it is essential that the results of laboratory experiments be applied to human beings to further scientific knowledge and to help suffering humanity, the World Medical Association has prepared the following recommendations as a guide to every physician in biomedical research involving human subjects. They should be kept under review in the future. It must be stressed that the standards as drafted are only a guide to physicians all over the world. Physicians are not relieved from criminal, civil and ethical responsibilities under the laws of their own countries.

I. BASIC PRINCIPLES

1. Biomedical research involving human subjects must conform to generally accepted scientific principles and should be based on adequately performed laboratory and animal experimentation and on a thorough knowledge of the scientific literature.
2. The design and performance of each experimental procedure involving human subjects should be clearly formulated in an experimental protocol which should be transmitted to a specially appointed independent committee for consideration, comment and guidance.
3. Biomedical research involving human subjects should be conducted only by scientifically qualified persons and under the supervision of a clinically competent medical person. The responsibility for the human subject must always rest with a medically qualified person and never rest on the

subject of the research, even though the subject has given his or her consent.

4. Biomedical research involving human subjects cannot legitimately be carried out unless the importance of the objective is in proportion to the inherent risk to the subject.

5. Every biomedical research project involving human subjects should be preceded by careful assessment of predictable risks in comparison with foreseeable benefits to the subject or to others. Concern for the interests of the subject must always prevail over the interest of science and society.

6. The right of the research subject to safeguard his or her integrity must always be respected. Every precaution should be taken to respect the privacy of the subject and to minimize the impact of the study on the subject's physical and mental integrity and on the personality of the subject.

7. Physicians should abstain from engaging in research projects involving human subjects unless they are satisfied that the hazards involved are believed to be predictable. Physicians should cease any investigation if the hazards are found to outweigh the potential benefits.

8. In publication of the results of his or her research, the physician is obliged to preserve the accuracy of the results. Reports of experimentation not in accordance with the principles laid down in this Declaration should not be accepted for publication.

9. In any research on human beings, each potential subject must be adequately informed of the aims, methods, anticipated benefits and potential hazards of the study and the discomfort it may entail. He or she should be informed that he or she is at liberty to abstain from participation in the study and that he or she is free to withdraw his or her consent to participation at any time. The doctor should then obtain the subject's freely-given informed consent, preferably in writing.

10. When obtaining informed consent for the research project the physician should be particularly cautious if the subject is in a dependent relationship to him or her or may consent under duress. In that case the informed consent should be obtained by a physician who is not engaged in the investi-

gation and who is completely independent of this official relationship.

11. In case of legal incompetence, informed consent should be obtained from the legal guardian in accordance with national legislation. Where physical or mental incapacity makes it impossible to obtain informed consent, or when the subject is a minor, permission from the responsible relative replaces that of the subject in accordance with national legislation.

    Whenever the minor child is in fact able to give a consent, the minor's consent must be obtained in addition to the consent of the minor's legal guardian.

12. The research protocol should always contain a statement of the ethical considerations involved and should indicate that the principles enunciated in the present Declaration are complied with.

II. MEDICAL RESEARCH COMBINED WITH PROFESSIONAL CARE (CLINICAL RESEARCH)

1. In the treatment of the sick person, the physician must be free to use a new diagnostic and therapeutic measure, if in his or her judgment it offers hope of saving life, reestablishing health or alleviating suffering.

2. The potential benefits, hazards and discomfort of a new method should be weighed against the advantages of the best current diagnostic and therapeutic methods.

3. In any medical study, every patient—including those of a control group, if any—should be assured of the best proven diagnostic and therapeutic method.

4. The refusal of the patient to participate in a study must never interfere with the physician-patient relationship.

5. If the doctor considers it essential not to obtain informed consent, the specific reasons for this proposal should be stated in the experimental protocol for transmission to the independent committee.[1,2]

6. The physician can combine medical research with professional care, the objective being the acquisition of new medical knowledge, only to the extent that medical re-

search is justified by its potential diagnostic or therapeutic value for the patient.

III. NONTHERAPEUTIC BIOMEDICAL RESEARCH INVOLVING HUMAN SUBJECTS (NON-CLINICAL BIOMEDICAL RESEARCH)

1. In the purely scientific application of medical research carried out on a human being, it is the duty of the physician to remain the protector of the life and health of that person on whom biomedical research is being carried out.
2. The subjects should be volunteers — either healthy persons or patients for whom the experimental design is not related to the patient's illness.
3. The investigator or the investigating team should discontinue the research if in his/her or their judgement it may, if continued, be harmful to the individual.
4. In research on man, the interest of science and society should never take precedence over considerations related to the wellbeing of the subject.

Index

*For Product Safety Concerns and Information please contact
our EU representative GPSR@taylorandfrancis.com Taylor & Francis
Verlag GmbH, Kaufingerstraße 24, 80331 München, Germany*

T - #0028 - 270225 - C0 - 229/152/9 [11] - CB - 9780866567190 - Gloss Lamination